MW00511296

Selected Models

of

Practice

in

Geriatric Psychiatry

*A Task Force Report of the
American Psychiatric Association*

The American Psychiatric Association
Task Force on Models of Practice in Geriatric Psychiatry

Marion Zucker Goldstein, M.D. (Chair)
Christopher C. Colenda, M.D., M.P.H.
Gary J. Kennedy, M.D.
Hugo Van Dooren, M.D.
William Van Stone, M.D.
Donald P. Hay, M.D.
Joel Sadavoy, M.D.

Selected Models
of
Practice
in
Geriatric Psychiatry

A Task Force Report of the
American Psychiatric Association

Published by the
American Psychiatric Association
Washington, DC

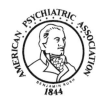

Note: The authors have worked to ensure that all information in this book concerning drug dosages, schedules, and routes of administration is accurate as of the time of publication and consistent with standards set by the U.S. Food and Drug Administration and the general medical community. As medical research and practice advance, however, therapeutic standards may change. For this reason and because human and mechanical errors sometimes occur, we recommend that readers follow the advice of a physician who is directly involved in their care or the care of a member of their family.

The findings, opinions, and conclusions of this report do not necessarily represent the views of the officers, trustees, all members of the task force, or all members of the American Psychiatric Association. The views expressed are those of the authors of the individual chapters. Task force reports are considered a substantive contribution of the ongoing analysis and evaluation of problems, programs, issues, and practices in a given area of concern.

Copyright © 1993 American Psychiatric Association
ALL RIGHTS RESERVED
Manufactured in the United States of America on acid-free paper
First Edition
96 95 94 93   4 3 2 1

American Psychiatric Association
1400 K Street, N.W., Washington, DC   20005

Library of Congress Cataloging-in-Publication Data
American Psychiatric Association. Task Force on Models of Practice in
  Geriatric Psychiatry.
    Selected models of practice in geriatric psychiatry : a Task Force
  report of the American Psychiatric Association. — 1st ed.
      p.   cm.
    Includes bibliographical references and index.
    ISBN 0-89042-239-7 (alk. paper)
      1. Geriatric psychiatry—Practice—United States.   2. Geriatric
  psychiatry—Practice.   I. Title.
      [DNLM: 2. Geriatric Psychiatry—organization & administration.
  2. Models, Psychological.   WT 150 A512s]
  RC451.4.A5A5   1993
  618.97'689'00973—dc20
  DNLM/DLC
  for Library of Congress   92-48940
                                                                  CIP

British Library Cataloguing in Publication Data
A CIP record is available from the British Library.

Acknowledgments and Support

The Task Force wishes to acknowledge the generous gift of time and expertise given to this report by Sanford Finkel, M.D.; Howard H. Goldman, M.D.; James A. Greene, M.D.; Linda Hay, Ph.D.; Gabe J. Maletta, M.D.; Rick A. Martinez, M.D.; Pat McKegney, M.D.; Edwin J. Olsen, M.D.; Kimberly A. Sherrill, M.D., M.P.H.; and Gary W. Small, M.D. The cooperation of Tom Dial, Ph.D.; David B. Larson, M.D., M.S.P.H.; John Lyons, Ph.D.; and Harold Alan Pincus, M.D., has been invaluable in enabling us to add a chapter on professional profiles of psychiatrists who attend to the mental health of our elderly population.

Publication of this report was made possible, in part, by an educational grant from Sandoz Pharmaceutical Company.

Table of Contents

Introduction

The provision of mental health care for the elderly may occur in many different settings and may be undertaken by professionals trained in a variety of disciplines. Where mental health services and professionals are available to them, the elderly often do not utilize mental health services at the same rate as other groups in our population. Thus, elders with mental disorders often remain undiagnosed and untreated. The reasons many older persons do not seek care are manyfold. The stigma of mental illness is still a major barrier to care for this population. Equally, treatment may be precluded because depression, confusion, or lost cognitive capacity may be thought to be part of "normal" aging processes. Further, many elderly people fall between the cracks of poorly coordinated health and social service programs. The history of a $250 annual ceiling on Medicare outpatient mental health services for many years, followed by a cap of $1,100 per year, which was finally removed, certainly delayed any incentive for outpatient mental health care for the elderly. The 50% copayment for outpatient mental health services posed a major disincentive to treatment of mental disorders of Medicare recipients. Introduction of Evaluation/Management (E/M) Current Procedural Terminology (CPT) codes through the Resource Based Relative Value Scale (RBRVS) in January 1992 with 20% copayment for specialty services is as yet subject to regional variations in interpretations for applicability to psychiatric outpatient care.

As our population ages—with the ranks of those over the age of 65 expected to reach nearly 35 million by the turn of the century—the need for specialized geriatric physical and mental health care grows. Although the rapidly developing field of geriatric psychiatry has expanded broadly over the past few years, functioning primarily at the interface of physical and mental health care, its growth and that of geriatric treatment facilities will be outstripped by the growth of the population in need. In part, the inadequate numbers of specialized professionals in geriatric mental health care is the result of ageism.[1] Some of the problem may be attributed to the complexities in treatment of the elderly, in which particular attention must be paid to the interrelationships of chronic physical disease and mental disorders. Certainly, part of the problem is the direct result of financial disincentives in Medicare and Medicaid reimbursement that discourage participation by many psychiatrists. The availability of community-based comprehensive mental health services for mentally ill people of all ages, though an economically prudent response to high-cost institutional care, has so far lacked consistent implementation. We know that although the census of state mental hospitals has declined drastically during the past decade and a half (Fogel et al. in press) and waiting lists for nursing homes are inordinately long (Borson et al. 1989), the bulk of funds have not followed the patient into the community. Complexity of care, increasing workload, and inadequate funding are major disincentives to the initiation and growth of programs.

One challenge for geriatric psychiatry is to expand the as yet limited number of psychiatric treatment services that can provide the comprehensive care required by both older persons with multiple medical problems and their families. Such services ideally should be placed strategically at the cutting edge of science, allowing new research discoveries to be translated rapidly into clinical practice. Over the past decade, in an effort both to respond to this challenge and to meet the future needs of our aging society, a variety of innovative approaches have been implemented in the United States and abroad.

Another challenge for geriatric psychiatry is to educate and enlighten both legislators and the public to diminish stigma and eliminate discriminatory reimbursement policies.

The Role of the Task Force

To help identify and describe innovative programs that represent models to be emulated in the field, the American Psychiatric Association (APA) established the

---

[1]Butler (1975) has suggested that many physicians and other health-care professionals consciously choose to avoid working with the elderly for what are actually subconscious reasons. They fear their own mortality and do not wish to face it daily by working with elderly patients. Many avoid working with older people who have chronic disorders. These physicians find greater fulfillment in working with those with extended lifetimes before them, managing acute rather than chronic disease.

Task Force on Models of Practice in Geriatric Psychiatry in May 1989. Its charge was to "produce a document and/or other educational materials to provide practical information to APA members, other service providers, health-care planners, legislators, and others interested in expanding services in this area."

The document the Task Force produced was to delineate the various settings in which psychiatrists treat the elderly, and describe the targeting and identification of patients, clinical problems addressed, approaches to treatment, physical plant and staffing requirements, administrative issues, and reimbursement sources for each setting. Practical approaches to the practice of geriatric psychiatry in other countries and the special service delivery needs of ethnic minority patients were also to be addressed.

The Task Force began its work in September 1989 by identifying specific treatment settings in which geriatric psychiatry is practiced. Task Force members agreed to develop materials related to one or more of those settings, gathering information based on the current literature, conversations with psychiatric leaders in the particular settings, and personal experience. A call for submissions of Models of Practice in Geriatric Psychiatry in *Psychiatric News* did not produce any submissions. Sanford Finkel, M.D., President of the International Psychogeriatric Association, reviewed cross-national perspectives, and Howard H. Goldman, M.D., reviewed reimbursement issues.

A historical perspective was obtained by Task Force review of the Joint Information Service (APA and Mental Health Association) publication, *Creative Mental Health Services for the Elderly* (Glasscote et al. 1977), and of an unpublished analysis of the 1982 APA Professional Activities Survey, *Psychiatry and the Elderly: Differences in Practitioner Characteristics* (Blalock and Dial 1982). Members of the American Association for Geriatric Psychiatry were helpful in identifying successful programs. Psychiatrists active in the International Psychogeriatric Association supplied overviews on the status of geriatric psychiatry in various countries. A Joint Report of the Royal College of Physicians of London and the Royal College of Psychiatrists, *Care of Elderly People with Mental Illness: Specialist Services and Medical Training* (Royal College of Physicians and Royal College of Psychiatrists 1989), served as a valuable guide for concise presentation of complex issues in service delivery for the elderly.

As noted in the Joint Information Service publication (Glasscote et al. 1977), treatment delivery models are generally created by innovative creative psychiatrists and sustained by a combination of public and private funds. To be a model, a health-care delivery program

1. Enjoys consumer, family, community, and provider satisfaction;
2. Has been proven efficacious by well-defined outcome parameters;

3. Experiences financial survival, solvency, and perpetuity; and
4. Is flexible and adaptive to varying and growing needs.

In practice, comprehensive criteria of this nature are rarely studied systematically in service settings. When available, outcome criteria of particular programs have been included in this report. No meta-analytic or other systematic review of service outcome in geriatric psychiatry has been undertaken as yet. Model building in this theoretical area has yet to occur.

Settings chosen as the focus of this Task Force Report include

1. Consultation/liaison services in general hospitals and in comparison to consultation/liaison services in nursing homes;
2. Community mental health center services for the elderly, outreach, home health, day hospital, and respite care;
3. Psychiatric inpatient and outpatient services in the private sector (including discussion of university affiliation and managed care relationships);
4. The Veterans Administration mental health service system;
5. A continuity-of-care model from Canada; and
6. Programs developed in other countries.

Previously published Task Force Reports, developed by other components of the American Psychiatric Association's Council on Aging, have focused on long-term institutionalization of mentally ill elderly people in nursing homes (Borson et al. 1989), in state hospitals (Fogel et al. in press), and on the needs of mentally ill elderly people who are members of ethnic minorities (Sakauye et al. in press). Rather than refocus on these well-described areas of interest, this Task Force chose to examine settings not discussed in these prior reports. Where appropriate, however, the earlier reports are referenced.

The Task Force's goal is to provide a working document for clinicians, policymakers, and others engaged in developing working programs to meet the mental health needs of our aging population. By identifying and describing existing models of excellence in geriatric psychiatry practice, found in a variety of settings and geographic locations, the Task Force hopes to embolden others to use these as paradigms for future service system development.

Chapter 1

Consultation/Liaison Service Models

Although older adults (age 65+) represent 12% of the United States population, they account for more than 35% of the admissions to acute care beds in general hospitals. The average hospital stay of the older patient is as much as 30% longer than the stay of the younger patient (National Center for Health Statistics 1982). About 40%–50% of elderly patients hospitalized with a physical disorder have a diagnosable psychiatric disorder before hospital discharge (Lipowski 1983). Psychiatrists working in the field of consultation/liaison (C/L) psychiatry work at this interface between physical and mental disorder, providing psychiatric intervention for medical/surgical patients who develop emotional disorders while hospitalized. Notwithstanding the increasing numbers of older persons seen in C/L psychiatry practice, little attention has been paid to the changing role of the C/L psychiatrist (Goldberg 1989). Lipowski (1983) was among the first to point out that the role of the C/L psychiatrist increasingly has been shifted toward geriatric care, making such psychiatrists de facto psychogeriatricians. He called specifically for broader geriatric education for C/L psychiatrists.

Studies that followed Lipowski's call to integrate C/L with geriatric psychiatry identified aspects of consultant knowledge and practice that were particularly relevant to the elderly (Perez et al. 1985; Popkin et al. 1984; Rosse et al. 1986; Ruskin 1985; Small and Fawzy 1988). Goldberg (1989) identified a number of areas in which the C/L psychiatrist must show geriatric expertise:

✦ The stress of hospitalization with its unfamiliar environments, complex evaluations, and uncertainties of treatment are more threatening for the elderly. Forced dependency, although temporary, may be overwhelming to a frail but previously independent older adult.

1

✦ The presence of multiple medical conditions and gender- and age-related increases in interindividual physiologic heterogeneity make it more difficult to minimize the risk of adverse reactions to medications. Diagnosis is similarly made more difficult by the multiplicity of ongoing treatments and conditions. The result, in part, is a more frequent finding of dementia, delirium, and affective disorders, with anxiety, somatic, or personality disorders seen less often.

✦ Both the severity and persistence of cognitive impairment may mislead well-intentioned primary care physicians and consultants as to the efficacy of psychiatric intervention in late life. Negative social and gender stereotypes and age-related biases catalogued by Butler (1975) also affect physician decisions, as noted in Kiloh's paper on pseudodementia (1961). However, the well-trained C/L psychiatrist has been shown to have a positive impact not only on the psychological well-being of hospitalized older patients but on their physical recovery as well (Strain et al. 1991).

✦ Interview techniques require modification to attend to the sensory impairments and social expectations of older persons. Auditory acuity in the higher frequencies is frequently degraded in late life. To compensate, the consultant should speak in lower tones, remain in full sight of the patient, and conduct the interview in as quiet an environment as possible. The social approach should be more deferential than familiar or casual. A collateral source of information (usually a family member or friend of the patient) is crucial both to give an objective view of the older patient's prior level of function and support as well as to minimize the burden of detail placed on the older primary informant. (We suggest that family engagement also allows the consultant to assess caregiver burden; to assess potential or actual abuse, neglect, or exploitation; to educate the family about the patient's condition; and to reinforce therapeutic recommendations.)

✦ Finally, a thorough grounding in the biological determinants of mental impairment, age- and gender-related changes in physiology, and expertise in psychopharmacology are essential. Also, the consultant must be knowledgeable in the assessment of the person's capacity to make health-care decisions.

We can add to Goldberg's areas of needed geriatric expertise a knowledge of state laws on health-care proxy assignments, living wills, the federally mandated Patient Self-Determination Act, and state elder abuse reporting laws.

However, the well-trained C/L psychiatrist has been shown to have a positive impact not only on the psychological well-being of hospitalized older patients but on their physical recovery as well (Strain et al. 1991).

Theoretical Models

Greenhill has proposed a number of models of methods through which mental health services and training can be delivered on medical and surgical units (Greenhill 1979; Greenhill and Kilgore 1950). In the *consultation model,* the primary physician refers the patient for psychiatric evaluation. This model forms the basis for other variations. In the *liaison model,* a consulting psychiatric service is assigned to work with patients and physicians from specific hospital units designated by the parent department. The *milieu model* extends the liaison model to encompass the social psychology of patient care. Although greater collaboration with social work and nursing staff results, the primary physician remains responsible for identification and triage of patients even though the psychiatrist is an identified "insider" in the ward culture (Mohl 1979). The *critical care model* is a subset of the milieu model in which the liaison with the psychiatrist is forged by an intensive care unit rather than the parent department. In the *biological psychiatry model,* a derivative of the consultation model, the psychiatrist relies predominantly on expertise in neurosciences and psychopharmacology, with less emphasis on psychodynamics and social psychology.

In the *integral model,* favored by Greenhill, any member of the health-care team may request psychiatric consultation. The distinguishing characteristic of the integral model is a focus on primary prevention by early identification of patients who are at high risk for episodes of mental illness or difficulty in collaborating with treatment. These patients are characterized by certain conditions (e.g., substance abuse), need for specific medical procedures (e.g., hemodialysis), advanced age, or disadvantaged ethnic or other minority status. This integral model also maintains an auditing procedure to determine the appropriateness of a request for and the provision of psychiatric C/L services.

Empirical Models

Strain and colleagues (1985) have identified empirical mental health training models for primary care physicians in which C/L psychiatrists play a significant role. Similarly, McKegney and Schwartz (1986) have described the organizational and treatment issues that arise between C/L psychiatry and the emerging field of behavioral medicine. Both reports emphasize the diversity and the limitations that arise out of the "local politics" under which the programs evolved. However, the effectiveness of the programs—whether the focus is patient care, clinical training, or research—depends on strong leadership, mutually perceived needs, and realistically defined goals. As with any collaborative effort, the smaller, more specialized component of the program (i.e., mental health) is vulnerable to the preferences and personalities of the larger.

Gallagher and colleagues (1990) describe both the promise and problems in the development of a Behavioral Medicine Service at the University of Vermont College of Medicine. Although the biopsychosocial diagnostic net espoused by Gallagher and colleagues is conceptually well suited to the problems of the elderly, only 9 of 678 individuals referred to this service were found to have an organic mental syndrome. Thus, despite conceptual readiness, not all C/L and behavioral medicine services will be psychogeriatric as well.

Nursing Home Consultation/Liaison Services

Case Study

Following a massive stroke, Mr. A., a 67-year-old executive, was saved as the result of extensive neurosurgery; nonetheless, he was left severely disabled. When he was admitted to a nursing home after recovery from surgery in the acute care general hospital, staff found his wife to be both clinging and depressed; his children were angry and demanding. The family believed the nursing home staff to be indifferent to Mr. A.'s rehabilitation potential, a scenario that had been played out just weeks before in the general hospital. Staff considered the family's request that Mr. A. be evaluated for depression to be little more than an exercise in denial of his inevitable decline. Nonetheless, staff agreed to hold a conference with a psychiatric consultant, if for no other reason than to help the family adjust to Mr. A.'s continued disability.

During the conference, Mrs. A. admitted to being overwhelmed by her husband's disabilities. His daughter wondered why aggressive rehabilitation was not being attempted for her father. The psychiatric consultant acknowledged the differences of opinion about Mr. A.'s prognosis, but suggested that implementation of a trial of physical therapy would not compromise either side in the dispute. The consultant also noted that although Mr. A. appeared not to be depressed, his somnolence might be related to his medication regimen—a combination of phenobarbital and phenytoin prescribed for seizure prophylaxis. These medications had been prescribed by the family physician whom Mr. A. had trusted for many years. When the phenobarbital was discontinued, Mr. A. became more active in physical therapy. Nonetheless, some obvious deficits in motor activity remained. During the course of Mr. A.'s rehabilitation, social work staff provided support to his wife.

Eight months after the stroke, Mr. A. walked out of the facility to return home to his family, who would care for him with the assistance of part-time in-home help. The psychiatric consultant in this case was a fellowship-trained geriatric psychiatrist; the intervention was typical of the kind provided when nursing home C/L services are available.

The recent requirements mandated by Congress for nursing homes include the assurance that the resident is free from the threat of chemical or physical restraints and the requirement that patients be prescreened to determine the need for psychiatric care. Historically, while including many mentally ill residents in their census, nursing homes have not had sufficient numbers of psychiatrists (and more specifically, geriatric psychiatrists) on staff or on call to meet those residents' needs (Borson et al. 1989). Data from empirical studies indicate that the models of care described in the earliest C/L literature may guide current development of psychiatric services in nursing homes.

Borson and colleagues (1987) have estimated that less than 1% of elderly nursing home residents who might benefit from psychiatric assessment and intervention actually receive such services. Even when consultations are provided, they may differ radically from the interventions undertaken by a hospital-based C/L service. Lippert and colleagues (1990) compared the characteristics of psychiatric consultations for elderly patients in a general hospital with those found in consultations provided in an affiliated nursing home. Several important differences were identified. General hospital consultations more frequently were for acute situations, requiring contact with other physicians, necessitating a substantial number of visits in the 2 weeks immediately following the initial patient contact, and using a variety of psychotherapeutic and pharmacotherapeutic interventions. In contrast, nursing home consultations were more frequently requested in the wake of patient behavior difficulties for which the facility sought diagnostic answers, and entailed substantial contact with nurses and other nonphysician health-care professionals. Dementia was diagnosed in 70% of the nursing home consultations and 27% of the general hospital consultations (Lippert et al. 1990). Psychiatric C/L is an essential nursing home service, particularly considering the heterogeneous and complex manifestations of dementia and the lack of mental health training of most nursing home staff.

Based on their personal experience with nursing home residents, Bienenfeld and Wheeler (1989) emphasize the need for a C/L model for nursing homes. When working with residents referred to their private practices from a nursing home, Bienenfeld and Wheeler found that the staff accompanying the resident knew little about the patient, were unable to provide relevant collateral information, and did not perceive themselves as therapeutic agents. Moreover, the authors reasoned that this absence of information on the part of the staff accompanying the patient represented only the tip of the iceberg. In response, the authors switched to an on-site evaluation of nursing home patients, followed by a case conference scheduled to bridge the nursing staff's change of shift. They also found it useful to establish ongoing contact with administrative staff to ensure the integration of clinical and administrative interests in the care of the residents seen in C/L. The psychiatrists were paid for their C/L services directly by the nursing facility; the nursing home did the billing and was reimbursed by Medicare (Part B). Because Bienenfeld and Wheeler carefully documented the services they rendered, the nursing home experienced an increase in its Medicaid allotment (Bienenfeld and Wheeler 1989)—a unique local event with no known replications.

Little is known of the relative efficacy of temporarily transferring mentally ill or otherwise disruptive nursing home patients to acute care geriatric psychiatry units in general hospitals or to freestanding psychiatric hospitals. However, we do know that patients with cognitive impairments find it difficult to adapt to new environments. We also know that the frail elderly, as a class, are exceptionally vulnerable to disorientation due to relocation. Both of these factors suggest that greater use of C/L psychiatry services for nursing home patients would be beneficial.

Consultation/Liaison Reimbursement Issues

The requests for C/L psychiatric care come primarily from medicine, surgery, and other specialties. For the most part, such services are rendered in general hospital settings. During the course of preparation of this report, until January 1992, a psychiatric consultation was reimbursed by Medicare on a one-time-only basis; a limited number of follow-up visits could be charged as psychotherapy without regard to the psychiatrist's liaison activities or interactions with a patient's family. A report containing either the medical license number or other identification of the referring physician had to be submitted to Medicare if an "extended" consultation by a C/L psychiatrist was to be reimbursed under Part B of the Medicare insurance program. These financial constraints limited the extent to which comprehensive mental health care was available for physically ill elderly patients in a general hospital that lacked either salaried medical staff or medical school affiliation. The capacity of psychiatric services to offset the cost of inpatient surgery has now been demonstrated (Strain et al. 1991). Yet hospital administrators often do not recognize the benefits of adding C/L psychiatrists to the hospital's salaried staff.

If the liaison function is not maintained over time and if a consistent model is not followed, one-time psychiatric consultations for physically ill patients may generate valuable recommendations that receive no follow-up attention. For a psychiatric C/L service to be successful and effective, the support of the hospital administration is critical. Equally important is ongoing assistance to maintain patient records that include patient and caregiver profiles, diagnostic assessments, recommendations made, recommendations followed, and effectiveness of those recommendations. Such record keeping not only helps track individual patients but also allows the C/L service to study itself, facilitating both service growth and resident and student education and training. These are vital, time-consuming C/L activities to which reimbursement, so far, has not been committed.

Although the number of elderly patients seen by psychiatrists on consultation services is high, opportunities for assessment, treatment, and well-planned follow-up after discharge from the hospital are limited as the result of Diagnostic Related Group (DRG) limitations on hospital stays and concomitant economic constraints on both providers and patients for follow-up outpatient or in-home mental health services.

Three developments occurring between preparation and publication of this report are likely to have an impact on C/L reimbursements within both hospital and nursing home that is significant but difficult to predict. Legislation has been introduced in the U.S. Senate to make Medicare payments for psychiatric care provided in a nursing facility comparable to that provided to hospital inpatients. Specifically, reimbursement rates for nursing home services would be raised to the 80-20 Medicare/copayment ratio. If enacted, this legislation would improve the recoverable costs of nursing home psychiatric services. Furthermore, the Health Care Financing Administration (HCFA) has circulated rules that would bundle outpatient imaging, laboratory, equipment (e.g., wheelchairs), and consultant fees following a hospital stay. In effect, the hospital would assume responsibility for containing costs allowed for DRG conditions incurred during the hospital stay and after discharge as well.

Finally, the Resource Based Relative Value Scale (RBRVS) and procedural codes emerging as this report goes to press will have considerable effect on consultation services. The range of services that psychiatric consultants can now bill has been expanded. However, the manner in which the HCFA and the regional insurance carriers interpret the Evaluation/Management codes and set reimbursement levels based on complexity of the consultation ultimately will determine the extent to which psychiatric services will expand. These latter matters are subject to much uncertainty at this time.

Chapter 2

Community-Based Models of Mental Health Services for the Elderly: Outreach and Respite Care Programs

As previously mentioned, elders are low utilizers of mental health services (Burns and Taube 1990). A variety of reasons have been offered to explain this finding, such as ageism, stigma, inadequate detection of mental health problems, language barriers, poorly coordinated health and social services, and reimbursement disincentives (Lebowitz et al. 1987). The estimated mental health services need by elderly patients is approximately 7.8% (Shapiro et al. 1985). Unfortunately, only 4.9% of elderly people living in the community who are in need of treatment are actually receiving care; 2.5% of them receive care by the specialty mental health sector, while another 2.4% are treated in the general medical sector (Burns and Taube 1990).

The gap between the delivery of services and the need for services is compounded by poor detection rates, fragmentation of services, and excessive reliance on medications, especially in the general medical care sector. For example, although the recognition of mental disorders in the elderly by primary care physicians is considered an important task, studies consistently found problems in recognition, treatment, and referral of these patients by primary care physicians (German et al. 1987; Jencks 1985; Rapp et al. 1991; Schurman et al. 1985). Detection rates of mental disorders in the elderly by primary care physicians are consistently low—less than 10% in some studies (Rapp et al. 1991). In addition, these practitioners rely heavily on medication management for symptoms, and little time is devoted to counseling services (Burns and Taube 1990). It is understandable that primary care physicians may not have the time or expertise to counsel elderly patients with disabling emotional distress. But, it is disturbing and unclear why primary care physicians fail to refer these patients to mental health specialists more often. Some speculate that the failure to refer can be explained by physicians harboring attitudes that may trivialize disorders such as depression, anxiety, and early dementia as expected manifestations of old age. This speculation casts negative aspersions on busy primary care physicians that may not be justified. Other explanations yet untested probably account for these practice patterns.

The distribution of mental health services in the specialty mental health sector is an interesting counterpoint to those provided by the general medical care sector. Of the 2.5% community-based elderly who receive treatment from the specialty mental health sector, nearly 60% are treated by private psychiatrists, 10% are treated by clinical psychologists, and 12% by staff of community mental health centers (CMHC). The remaining 18% receive treatment from non-CMHC clinics, partial hospitalization programs, and the Department of Veterans Affairs (Burns and Taube 1990). Patients in the specialty mental health sector receive more counseling services than patients in the general medical care sector, but coordination of services may not be very efficient, especially as the severity of the primary psychiatric illness and medical comorbidities increases.

Coordination of services is vital if elderly patients are to be maintained in the community for as long as possible. But we have seen here, coordinated systems of care, such as CMHCs, are also underutilized by elderly people (Burns and Taube 1990). This trend is important, because insufficient numbers of private practitioners (whether in the general medical sector or specialty mental health sector) have the time, resources, or fiscal incentives to coordinate a wide array of services for these patients. The relatively low utilization of services provided by CMHCs by elderly patients may be attributable to the paucity of specialized geriatric staff at such facilities. More than one-third (281) of 645 CMHCs that are members of the National Council of Community Mental Health Centers reported that they served geriatric patients (Light et al. 1986); 56 of these identified themselves as specialized centers with specific geriatric services. Only 105 of CMHCs were found to include both specialized staff and service. Twenty-eight reported the presence of special services but no specialized staff; 16 reported the use of specialty staff used strictly in the provision of specialty geriatric services.

Most specialized CMHCs reported that they provided comprehensive physical examinations and maintained a variety of family related services, support/socialization groups, transportation services, and services for dementia patients and their families. Specialized CMHCs generally maintained linkages with senior citizen centers, home-based services, residential facilities, and nursing homes (Light et al. 1986). Of the 281 CMHCs that reported serving geriatric patients, 185 had established formal relationships with local Area Agencies on Aging (AAAs). These CMHCs reported the association with the AAAs led to instances of shared funding, service and educational program planning, and staff liaison. Not surprisingly, the percentage of patients over the age of 60 seen in these AAA-affiliated CMHCs is, on average, 31% higher than found in CMHCs without such affiliations (Lebowitz et al. 1987).

Case Management and Outreach Programs: Concepts and Practices

Understanding the service utilization trends in CMHCs that have specialized mental health services for geriatric patients from those that don't is important if attempts are to be made to improve utilization and accessibility of mental health services by the elderly. The evidence clearly suggests that coordinated services improve utilization. Given this finding, and the corresponding reasons offered as explanations for why the elderly don't use mental health services, what avenues are available to improve accessibility of care? One option is mental health outreach programs. These programs have been a relatively recent development in community mental health systems (Bush et al. 1990; Thompson et al. 1990). By and large these programs are designed to deal with difficult younger patients with persistent and severe mental illnesses who have fallen through the cracks of the community mental health support network. Model programs such as Assertive Continuous Care Teams (ACCT) in Madison, Wisconsin (Stein 1990) are multidisciplinary, set no time limits for patient involvement, are case management oriented, and when necessary deal with patients in their home environments.

"Case management" is important for outreach programs. It refers to maintaining a mentally ill person's emotional, physical, and social environment with the goal of facilitating community placement, survival, adaptation, and personal growth (Kantor 1989). Case management involves a variety of functions, including assessment, planning, linking, monitoring, and advocacy (Intagliata 1982; Kantor 1989). Kantor operationalizes the role of case manager into 13 different domains:

Initial Phase
1. Engagement
2. Assessment
3. Planning

Environmental Interventions
4. Linkage with community services
5. Consultation with families and other caregivers
6. Maintenance and expansion of social networks

7. Collaboration with physicians and hospitals
8. Advocacy

Patient Interventions
9. Intermittent individual psychotherapy
10. Training in independent living skills
11. Patient psychoeducation

Patient-Environment Interventions
12. Crisis intervention
13. Monitoring

Some have criticized the case management model on grounds of efficiency and efficacy (Franklin et al. 1987). But others have shown that health services utilization of chronic mentally ill adults who receive intensive community outreach services had significantly fewer hospital days, adhered to their treatment plans more often, and used fewer emergency services when compared to a control group of similar patients (Bush et al. 1990). Interestingly, case management has been adopted by the general medical care sector and social service agencies to provide long-term community-based care to medically ill or disabled geriatric patients. These programs offer a spectrum of services from which the case manager can choose, in order to successfully maintain an "at-risk" elder in the community. The "menu" of services available to the older adult can range from "home-based sitters" and homemaker aides to nursing services, occupational and physical therapy, social services, Meals on Wheels, and in some cases, physician services. The key to service delivery is matching the patient's needs with available community resources.

Data bearing on the efficacy of outreach programs designed specifically for mentally ill elderly people are severely limited. Most studies have been anecdotal and descriptive in nature (Parish and Landsberg 1984; Reifler et al. 1982). Commentary about outreach programs for these patients advocates that a multidisciplinary team must be employed that can coordinate and access a variety of goods and services (Cohen 1991).

Thus, outreach by well-trained geriatric mental health practitioners appears critical if we are to ensure that community-based elderly people with mental illness are to be served appropriately, adequately, and cost-effectively. In contrast to many physical disorders in the older population, mental illness is not one for which treatment is routinely sought. Denial, fear, ageism, insufficient numbers of well-trained mental health care geriatricians—all conspire to limit access to care. Traditional community-based service delivery models must be reevaluated and redefined to meet this population's most urgent needs.

A Model Outreach and Treatment Program

Case Study

Ms. B., a 79-year-old widow, lives in her home of 45 years outside a major metropolitan city in the Midwest. Her two daughters and son left home to attend college and have since moved to other communities. Currently, one daughter, age 39 and divorced, has a sales job that requires her to travel extensively; the other daughter, age 35 and married with 2 children, is a homemaker in a town approximately 100 miles from her mother. Ms. B.'s son, age 33, married and a lawyer, lives in Los Angeles; since his father's death 4 years earlier, he has rarely seen his mother.

Immediately after the death of her husband, Ms. B. managed well. She remained active in her church and with a small circle of friends. However, approximately 2 years prior to contact with Outreach Services (a program supported by the regional community mental health center), friends noted that Ms. B. had become less involved in her church and social activities. During the Christmas holidays, she had become visibly confused and distraught at a church reception and left when the pastor tried to console her. Since that episode, friends rarely saw her in church; when her pastor came to call on her, she would not allow him into her home.

Increasingly, Ms. B. became isolated and suspicious. When her daughters came to visit, they found the house messy, dirty, and filled with daily newspapers. Both daughters were distressed and confronted their mother about her increasingly bizarre behavior. She dismissed their allegations.

Several months later, the daughter living closest to Ms. B. received an urgent phone call from the county assessor's office, claiming that her mother was delinquent in paying her taxes and had refused to receive registered letters. When the daughter arrived at her mother's home, she discovered that her mother refused to let anyone enter her home and had bolted all the doors. The daughter called the police and the emergency Outreach Crisis Intervention Team. After considerable negotiation, Ms. B. finally agreed to permit entry to her home. The police and the crisis team found her to be living in squalor. When she refused to be hospitalized voluntarily, the crisis team obtained an order permitting involuntary commitment.

During Ms. B.'s 3-week hospitalization, she was diagnosed with moderate dementia, including evidence of delusions. A regimen of low-dose neuroleptics ameliorated her paranoia, but increased the severity of her cognitive deficits. Ms. B. was extremely attached to her home and her daughter was reluctant to place her in a long-term care facility. Intensive outreach aftercare services were arranged by the treatment team. These services included weekly visits by Ms. B.'s psychiatric social worker–case manager to monitor the home environment, weekday homemaker services to help with cooking and self-care, weekend sitters, and transportation to and from the mental health clinic for medication checks. The family was referred to a local attorney to help establish durable power of attorney, guardianship, and living will procedures for Ms. B.

With the support received from the Outreach Services, Ms. B. was able to live successfully in her home for 3 more years. However, because of her increasing cognitive impairment and medical comorbidity, the program and the family agreed that Ms. B. should be placed in a nursing facility. Arrangements were managed with the assistance of Outreach Services.

The Spokane Community Mental Health Center's (SCMHC) Elderly Services Program stands as a model of how traditional mental health care services can be modified to provide the outreach and support necessary to meet the treatment needs of frail mentally ill elderly patients, as exemplified by the preceding case. This award-winning program, established in 1978, has sought to locate, identify, and provide care for mentally impaired elders residing in its catchment area (Raschko 1987). The Elderly Services program is actually two highly integrated programs: a telephone information and referral service and a multidisciplinary in-home evaluation, treatment, and case management team.

The well-publicized telephone information and referral service is staffed by three carefully trained telephone screeners and is targeted at "high functioning elder adults" who, at worst, are experiencing mild dysfunction. However, not all calls are simply for information or a casual referral. The screeners divert calls received after 5 P.M. or on weekends to the SCMHC crisis services. These crisis services provide 24-hour access to the second component of the Elderly Services program—in-home case management.

The goal of the in-home case management program is to maintain the independence of the elderly, to prevent premature or unnecessary institutionalization, and to improve the quality of life of this population at high risk for decline. In addition to referrals through the telephone information and referral service, a network of neighborhood "gatekeepers" identifies members of a high-risk population who have not sought needed care. The gatekeepers used in this program are nontraditional referral sources, and include a variety of individuals who may come in contact with the elderly on a routine basis: meter readers, repair personnel from home utility companies, property appraisers from the county assessor's office, trust officers and bank personnel, apartment managers, postal workers and letter carriers, fuel oil dealers, police officers, firefighters, sheriff's department employees, pharmacists, and ambulance drivers. These volunteers are trained by SCMHC to identify elderly people at high risk for mental disorders who are not likely to self-refer or who appear to lack either a formal or informal support network. Ongoing training programs are scheduled for these "gatekeepers"; communications are maintained with each "gatekeeper" about each referral made. The "gatekeeper program" now accounts for 40% of all referrals to the in-home case management program.

The multidisciplinary program staff includes 18 specialty trained case managers who carry primary responsibility for in-home intervention; four registered nurses and a social worker who serve as field supervisors; two psychiatrists who provide a combined 35 hours a week of in-home evaluation and treatment; a part-time family medicine resident from the University of Washington who is available 4 hours a week for in-home evaluation and treatment; and a master's degree social worker-program coordinator who functions under the direction of the program director.

Three case managers are assigned to each nurse field supervisor. The social worker field supervisor works with the remaining case managers who are graduate social work students engaged in their required field service through this program. The field supervisors carry out their supervision on a full-time basis: training the case managers, and accompanying them on home visits to assist in the assessment process and to help resolve difficult issues.

The average patient referred to the program is moderately to severely dysfunctional, isolated, and lacking in both community and family support. Losses in such areas as relationships; cognitive, emotional, and physical health; and property and familiar surroundings have contributed to the patient's functional decline. While in need of care, the typical elder identified by an SCMHC "gatekeeper" is distrustful of interventions, particularly by formal agencies because agency involvement might lead to removal from the home to nursing home placement, and further insults to continued autonomy. Fear, shame, and suspicion increase isolation and resistance to efforts to help.

After initial referral by either the "gatekeeper" or the telephone service, a case manager and a field supervisor are assigned to undertake an initial in-home functional assessment of the patient. One of their most important roles is to establish a positive trusting relationship with the elderly person. Other staff, such as a psychiatrist or the family medicine resident, may accompany the case manager on subsequent home visits for further evaluation and treatment.

A detailed service and treatment plan is written for each patient; it includes detailed information regarding the patient's physical, mental, socioeconomic, and environmental conditions. Special notes are made regarding medication monitoring requirements. Family and other individuals in the patient's support network are contacted. When appropriate, family conferences are convened. In addition to the provision of health care, a host of preventive, supportive, and rehabilitative in-home services are available through the SCMHC's relationship with the Eastern Washington Area Agency on Aging. These services include chore/homemaker services, visiting nurses, day health and day-care programs, home delivered meals, and respite care.

A particularly important aspect of this model is its primary ongoing case responsibility for all persons admitted to the program. Forty-nine percent of patients have been officially terminated after long periods of stabilization, 20% because of death, 12% after placement in a long-term care facility, 11% due to relocation, and the remaining 8% for a variety of other reasons. Yet, even after termination, the patient is followed either by telephone or through the in-home supportive network. If the patient has required hospitalization, the case manager continues the contact, participating, as appropriate, in outplacement to the community. In this way, the patient never falls through the cracks of the system; he or she is never passed from agency to agency depending on his or her needs for care.

The Holy Family Hospital's adult day program, a supportive and rehabilitative program, receives 64% of its referrals from the "Elderly Services" program.

In 1986, the Spokane program (SCMHC) served 538 patients, 62% women, 38% men; 5% were also minority elderly, who constitute 1.5% of the total 370,000 population of Spokane County. The 538 elderly presented various problems: physical illness (71%), social isolation (69%), personal care/ADL[1] problems (62%), depression (56%), environmental/social stress (67%), denial of illness or problem (60%), and memory impairment (59%). Only 5% of patients in the program had received prior outpatient or inpatient psychiatric care. By 1990, the case load had increased to 787. In 1978, the elderly constituted only 4% of the total number of patients seen by the SCMHC. In 1987, that percentage had risen to 22%; by 1990, it increased to 26%. Before 1980, Spokane County, as with so many other areas in the country, had a critical shortage of nursing home beds. Though the number of nursing home beds has not increased appreciably, there has been no shortage during the last 5 years of this program's operation. The suicide rate among the over-60 population in Spokane County has decreased from 33 per 100,000 to 19 per 100,000 over a 10-year period. Though suicide prevention services were available before the inception of the "Elder Services" program, they were not utilized by this high-risk group.

---

[1]ADL, or activities of daily living, includes a constellation of activities that are critical to self-care and independent living, such as toileting, feeding, dressing, shopping, and traveling by public conveyance. Limitations in ADL vary with physical and mental disability and are an important indicator of the ability to live independently.

Sixty percent of the financial support for operating costs of the Spokane Outreach Program has been provided by the Eastern Washington Area Agency on Aging. The remaining 40% comes from the Washington State Mental Health Grant-in-Aid and the National Institute of Drug Abuse. The National Institute of Mental Health has supported a practicum program for graduate social work students from Eastern Washington University who participate in the project. Of its $1.4-million budget, $1.1 million supports in-home evaluation and $300,000 underwrites both the telephone information and referral program and "gate-keeper" training.

Though the project has not been the subject of formal outcome, cost-effectiveness, or efficacy studies, this intensive case management outreach program designed to help elderly access needed mental health services not only makes sense intuitively, but also has demonstrated its effectiveness through the patients it has reached and helped as evidenced by the foregoing incidental findings. As a further tribute to its success as a model, a neighboring county has developed a similar program with several of its components coordinated with the existing Spokane County model. It is quite apparent that this or a similar system increases the utilization of community mental health services by the elderly.

A Model Dementia Care and Respite Service Program

Adult day programs and related services, such as respite care, are gradually becoming recognized as important new alternatives to institutional care for elderly patients with dementia. In August 1988, the Dementia Care and Respite Services Program (DCRS) demonstration project was created through a joint venture by the Robert Wood Johnson Foundation, the Administration on Aging, and the Alzheimer's Association. The DCRS is the first national project for adult day programs and, as such, is playing a major role in disseminating information about this approach to community-based care. Nineteen sites across 14 states nationwide were chosen from a pool of 283 applicants for this demonstration. Some of the chosen sites are freestanding centers; others were affiliated with nursing homes, senior centers or community agencies, medical centers, or city governments. Two are consortia of community-based organizations.

The articulated goals of each of the DCRS programs are to:

✦ Develop mechanisms to organize and finance services, with the aim of sustaining the Center over time;

✦ Develop or refine dementia-specific day treatment programs;

✦ Identify, through market research, other types of in-home and community-based respite care desired by caregivers;

✦ Develop a case-coordinated plan for each participant and caregiver to ensure access to needed services, whether provided by the Center or through referral to other agencies;

✦ Maintain linkages with community health and social services agencies, including Area Agencies on Aging, Alzheimer's Association chapters, and other voluntary organizations concerned with dementia;

✦ Involve caregivers and participants in the development of the dementia care program;

✦ Provide or arrange for dementia-specific training for caregivers, volunteers, and workers providing respite care in the day center or in the home; and

✦ Maintain direct contact with diagnostic and treatment facilities to provide treatment for behavioral or physical problems encountered in either participants or their caregivers.

The 19 sites are utilizing their funding in a variety of ways. Some have planned to renovate existing physical space either to expand the capacity of an existing program or to establish a new dementia-specific program. Others are expanding the duration of the program's hours to include weeknights, weekends, or overnight respite. Still others are developing in-home respite services. The funding also supports the establishment of unique program elements by some of the sites. One location is developing a "drop-in" center; another uses volunteers to work one-on-one with the participants. A third site trains high school students as respite workers for the program. The project's emphasis on financial independence is intended to increase the stability of programs that traditionally have been dependent on grants and donations as their primary sources of support.

In keeping with the variety of programs represented, staffing patterns are equally variable, based in part on whether the site has adopted a social model or a day health model of operation. All of the programs utilized health care professionals—usually nurses or social workers—in some capacity. These professionals serve in key administrative or program positions. Many program staff have had specialized training in recreational or music therapy. Sites operating under a day health model frequently contract with physical therapists or occupational therapists to provide services to the participants. Almost all social and day health model programs utilize volunteers in a variety of capacities.

Early data gathered on the first 450 participants who have enrolled in the day center programs indicate that participants have moderate cognitive impairment, with an average Mini-Mental State Exam (Folstein et al. 1975) score of 13.4. The data are based on information obtained in caregiver interviews at the time of participant enrollment in the program. The average number of impairments in ADL in the participants is 3.8, suggesting that they required either "some assistance" or "total assistance." Table 1 details the levels of impairment found in these participants across six important activities of daily living. Table 2 specifies the

Table 1. Activities of daily living ($N = 450$)

	No assistance		Some assistance		Complete assistance	
	#	(%)	#	(%)	#	(%)
Eating	220	(49)	191	(43)	35	(8)
Walking	236	(53)	159	(36)	52	(11)
Toileting	197	(44)	175	(39)	75	(17)
Grooming	120	(27)	205	(46)	121	(27)
Dressing	106	(24)	208	(47)	131	(29)
Bathing	80	(18)	198	(44)	168	(38)

Table 2. Participant behavior problems ($N = 450$)

Behavior problem	#	(%)
Difficulty concentrating on task	304	(68)
Shows little initiative to start activity	300	(67)
Cannot be left alone; must be supervised	293	(65)
Loses or misplaces things	288	(64)
Has difficulty following simple directions	266	(59)
Asks same question over again	254	(56)
Has difficulty communicating wants	237	(53)
Takes little interest in activities	235	(52)
Becomes stubborn or uncooperative	230	(51)
Frequently appears depressed	204	(45)
Wakes caregiver at night	194	(43)
Fails to recognize family or friends	183	(41)
Denies or is unaware anything is wrong	171	(38)
Demands constant attention	162	(36)
Becomes verbally abusive	136	(30)
Reports seeing or hearing things	130	(29)
Engages in embarrassing behavior	111	(25)
Wanders away from home	103	(23)
Engages in dangerous behavior	85	(19)
Becomes combative	80	(18)

frequency with which patients present specific behavior problems. Other program results, such as financial data and marketing information, will be available at a later date.

Chapter 3

Private-Sector Dedicated Psychogeriatric Services

In the 1960s, Great Britain and other European nations led the way in the development of specialized treatment programs for elderly people with mental illness by establishing separate "geriatric rehabilitation" programs and geriatric medical/psychiatric units in general hospitals. In the United States, the need for such acute care units dedicated to the special assessment and treatment needs of the elderly with late life onset of psychopathology is only now being recognized. Increasing numbers of general hospitals and freestanding psychiatric hospitals are establishing such special care units. The goal of such geriatric psychiatry units is to assure state-of-the-art assessment, improve function, enhance autonomy, and improve quality of life by assuring that an appropriate formal and informal support network is available to the patient upon discharge. Although geriatric psychiatrists generally agree on the efficacy of such units, few formal outcome studies have been conducted to date (Koran 1985; Rubenstein et al. 1980, 1982a, 1982b; Young and Harsch 1980).

A number of major deterrents confront those seeking to implement psychogeriatric comprehensive inpatient, day hospital, and outpatient services in the United States. The low regional Medicare per diem hospital reimbursement rate is foremost among the deterrents. Inpatient care is reimbursed at a daily rate of $200 to $500; day hospitalization rates range from $24 to $55. These rates are not in keeping with the special architectural and staffing patterns required for the elderly. The 190-day lifetime limitation on Medicare reimbursement for inpatient care in freestanding psychiatric hospitals poses yet another barrier. For many patients requiring hospital-based outpatient treatment, the 50% Medicare copayment for psychiatric treatment stood as a further barrier. The 1-day deductible per episode of psychiatric hospitalization creates a hardship for many Medicare recipients.

Medically indigent individuals may be able to surmount this obstacle if they reside in states in which Medicaid will pay the patient's copayment rate. Overall

Medicaid reimbursement rates for inpatient and outpatient physician services vary widely from state to state. In most states, Medicaid coverage of psychiatric services is substantially below prevailing rates. Because state governments have discretionary power over the types of programs covered under Medicaid, programs not covered by Medicare can therefore be established without a fee-for-service option.

Private insurance poses similar problems for mentally ill elderly people in need of treatment. Although 99% of private health insurance policies cover general inpatient care and 94% provide coverage for outpatient treatment, differences arise in the coverage of treatment for mental disorders. Only 53% of private policies cover inpatient mental illness treatment costs in the same manner as other illnesses are covered; only 7% of private insurers provide coverage for outpatient psychiatric services at the same rate as other disorders (American Psychiatric Association 1985). Most often, psychiatric coverage has been subject to higher coinsurance rates, limits on charges per visit and numbers of visits, and ceilings on annual reimbursement rates (Gottlieb 1988). The federal government has enacted a law to standardize all Medicare supplemental (Medigap) insurance policies. Implementation is currently under consideration by the National Commissioners of Health Insurance. How this will affect the still-remaining 50% copayment for outpatient mental health care instead of 20% for other medical care Evaluation/Management Current Procedural Terminology codes remains to be seen.

Yet another financial consideration is the fact that federally qualified health maintenance organizations (HMOs) that contract directly with Medicare are more likely to encourage outpatient primary care. Referral to specialists is often limited through the use of primary care "gatekeepers" (the term's usage here is not to be confused with its usage in outreach programs). In many instances, the HMO will contract with psychologists and social workers in lieu of psychiatrists. This may limit access to medical/mental health assessments, use of medications, or other somatic treatments that specialists may recommend and provide. In an HMO, the primary nonpsychiatric physician becomes the "gatekeeper" who potentially prevents rather than implements the outreach for specialized mental health services often needed by elderly patients and their families.

Other managed care methods have disrupted physician to physician referrals by establishing a limited panel of specialists of their choice and having a person in charge of their hot line decide where and to whom the patient participant should be referred.

Many of these and other aspects of the risks and benefits of establishing geriatric psychiatry inpatient units in general hospitals have been described by various authors who have struggled with these problems over the past decade (Barsa et al. 1985; Berger and King 1990; Billig and Leibenluft 1987; Cohen 1989; Conwell et al. 1989; Ford et al. 1980; Greene and Asp 1986; Schwartz et al. 1980).

Inpatient Psychogeriatric Unit Models

Two models of care that have been received with considerable enthusiasm have been described to the Task Force by their developers. Each involves significant collaboration among hospital administrators, fiscal officers, regional Medicare agencies, commercial insurers, local nursing homes, and geriatric psychiatrists. Such collaboration has been found to be critical to both development of and ongoing vitality of such programs.

Case Study: Senior Health Center—Health Corporation of America (HCA) Park West (Knoxville, Tennessee)

Mr. C., a 64-year-old married man, was admitted with symptoms including confusion, memory loss, crying spells, difficulty concentrating, and a preoccupation that "agents were following [him]." A psychiatric evaluation, including a dementia work-up, determined a diagnosis of major depression with delusions; all laboratory studies and X rays were within normal limits. Combination antidepressant and neuroleptic medications were initiated in conjunction with milieu, group, and individual psychotherapy. Mr. C.'s family was educated by staff about the psychodynamics of depression and paranoia and given guidance for intervention.

During his hospitalization, Mr. C. continued to report paranoid thoughts but began to refer to them in the past tense. On admission, he had refused food and expressed passive suicidal thoughts; one week later, he responded favorably to these interventions. He was discharged with improved affect and denied suicidal ideation; he was then followed up as an outpatient.[1]

This model is a nine-bed geriatric psychiatric medical unit that was developed cooperatively by two privately funded organizations. The unit was designed to adhere to Diagnostic Related Group (DRG) guidelines for admission, treatment, and discharge. The focus of this "Senior Health Center" is on the evaluation and short-term treatment of patients usually over the age of 60 who have been diagnosed with mood and/or memory disorders. Admission criteria include a primary psychiatric diagnosis, absence of severe acute or chronic physical conditions, and

---

[1] Unfortunately, no mention was made of Mr. C.'s. insurance coverage. Readers should be cautioned about this particular case in light of the clinical facts presented. Major depression with psychosis often only responds to treatment after a minimum of 6 weeks of trials of various medications and often requires a course of electroconvulsive therapy (ECT) treatments to effect symptomatic relief and functional improvement.

mobility sufficient to permit participation in the unit's activities program. Each patient is followed by both a psychiatrist and another physician chosen to attend to the patient's physical disorders. Unit policy provides for admission by family practitioners, internists, and neurologists after psychiatric consultation by a psychiatrist on the hospital's staff.

Because the unit adheres to DRG limitations, its emphasis has been on immediate and comprehensive patient assessment. The assessment begins with a physical examination by the primary physician and a psychiatric examination, including careful evaluation for dementia. The psychiatric examination includes the Short Portable Mental Status Examination (SPMSE; Pfeiffer 1975) and the Short Psychiatric Evaluation Scale (SPES; Pfeiffer et al. 1980). Diagnostic determinations are made consistent with DSM-III-R diagnostic criteria (American Psychiatric Association 1987). A psychosocial assessment, designed to identify vulnerabilities in the patient's resident environment, includes social, economic, and functional assessments. When a patient is to be admitted, a series of laboratory tests are scheduled: complete blood count, urinalysis, chem 23 (a screening battery of 23 chemical measurements), rapid plasma reagent, thyroxine/thyroid-stimulating hormone, B_{12} and folate levels, electrocardiogram, electroencephalogram, chest X ray (posteroanterior and lateral), computed tomography scan of head (or magnetic resonance imaging), daily weight, daily standing and lying blood pressure, geriatric nutritional assessment, and activity level. The Social Services department is consulted for assistance in discharge planning, and a family assessment is scheduled.

During the course of hospitalization, the patient's physical disorders are followed daily by the designated nonpsychiatric physician; specialists are consulted on an as-needed basis. Assessment data are routinely updated in writing by all staff members, focusing on orientation, affect, behavior patterns (socialization, sleeping, nutrition, elimination), and response to psychotropic and other medications. Functional levels are assessed daily and self-care is encouraged as tolerated. Individual treatment plans, reflecting overall program goals, include treatment of depression and other affective disorders with minimal use of ECT; treatment of insomnia, anxiety, delusions, hallucinations and psychotic behaviors, wandering, agitation, irritability and hostility; promotion of feelings of self-esteem; memory retrieval; treatment of physical health problems, with a focus on physical and speech therapy as needed; joint planning for appropriate discharge care needs; and modifications to living situations as needed.

The communication of significant patient information and coordination of responsibilities among the multidisciplinary team's members are enhanced by semiweekly conferences focusing on goal-directed assessment, treatment, and discharge planning. The meetings are attended by the geriatric psychiatrist, his or her staff, a family liaison nurse, a nurse manager, and other physicians who are on the unit at the time. Relevant patient information is shared, each patient's treatment goals are identified, progress is evaluated, and specific responsibilities are assigned.

Though no formal outcome studies of the special unit have been conducted, retrospective chart review of the first 100 patients yielded interesting data. The patients' mean age was 75 (range 51–90 years of age); 57 were female and 43 male. The average length of stay was 9.5 days (range 2–24 days). The mean SPMSE score of 54 patients on admission was 5.7 and at discharge 5.6, whereas the mean SPES score of 49 patients was 5.4 on admission and 3.5 at discharge. On discharge, 90 patients lived at home with some help; 10 required nursing home placement. These trends invite well-designed studies of the effect of brief hospitalizations on cognition and affect. The assessment unit identified a combination of 80 previously undiagnosed mental and physical disorders among the 100 admitted patients, including cases of Alzheimer's disease, depression, pernicious anemia, carcinoma, multi-infarct disease, cardiovascular disease, respiratory disease/chronic obstructive pulmonary disease, renal and urinary tract disease, alcohol abuse, normal pressure hydrocephalus, dental abscess/malnutrition, Parkinson's disease, auditory problems, iron deficiency, hyperthyroidism, decubitus ulcer, bilateral inguinal hernia, hiatal hernia, gastritis, aneurysm of the abdominal aorta, and fracture of humoral head. The brevity of these hospitalizations limits the conditions for which it can be effective.

Case Study: A Model University-Private Sector Geriatric Service (Milwaukee, Wisconsin)

Mrs. D., a 78-year-old widow, was referred to the outpatient clinic by her daughter. She had experienced a loss of interest, insomnia, lack of appetite, and impaired function. Her daughter reported what appeared to be an emerging delusional system: her mother thought a cousin was substituting objects in her house with facsimiles. Contact was made with Mrs. D.'s internist, and medical records were reviewed. A diagnosis of major depression with delusions led to treatment with nortriptyline with gradual increase to therapeutic blood levels and thiothixene. After 6 months, the psychotic component of Mrs. D.'s illness abated, and the thiothixene was gradually discontinued. Unfortunately, her remission was only temporary, and antipsychotic medication was reinstituted.

Mrs. D. was seen biweekly in the outpatient clinic. The nurse clinician spent considerable time with her and her family, both in person and on the telephone. Mrs. D. registered numerous complaints including burning eyes, tingling legs, lightheadedness, nervousness, and anxiety. The combination of antidepressants and neuroleptics did not relieve her symptoms of depression with delusions. She withdrew from all activities and would not leave her apartment. A course of ECT was recommended. Following six unilateral ECT treatments, Mrs. D. did well for several months. A relapse led to a course of outpatient ECT maintenance, which alleviated her symptoms. She resumed her activities in the community. Close communications were maintained with Mrs. D.'s internist to assist in differentiating between physical pathology and somatization secondary to her depression.

The Medical College of Wisconsin, working with St. Mary's Hill Hospital, a private psychiatric facility, has developed a division of geriatric psychiatry. The program is intended to provide a user-friendly system for both patient and provider of care, in which private psychiatrists can diagnose and treat their geriatric patients. The challenge for the partnership was to create a dedicated specialty staff able to bring state-of-the-art clinical care to the program. The program itself provides a multiplicity of services including liaison with all facilities and hospital and community resources that have a use for geriatric mental health services. Referrals to the program are made by family practitioners, internists, psychiatrists, mental health specialists, nursing home staff, social service agencies, and others who are aware of the program.

As mentioned previously, the fiscal solvency of such programs for the elderly has been questioned by many hospitals. St. Mary's Hill Hospital received capital improvement funds from its parent corporation to make extensive renovations to the facility. Because the hospital's administration recognized the program's need for both inpatient and outpatient services, revenues generated by both inpatient bed occupancy and outpatient fee-for-service charges were used to underwrite a portion of the program staff's salaries. By combining revenues from these two sources, decisions regarding the nature and locus of treatment were driven by sound clinical judgment and not only by fiscal considerations.

The geriatric psychiatry program utilizes one entire floor of the hospital. The 20-bed inpatient unit includes 6 beds for independent functioning patients and 14 beds for patients who require extensive care. The unit was designed by a cadre of professionals expert in the special environmental needs of the elderly. Thus, the walls are painted in lively colors; higher wattage lighting was installed. Handrails and mirrors were placed in suitable locations; the environment is wheelchair accessible. The unit is staffed by nurses, nurse's aides, an occupational therapist, a social worker, and a nurse clinician, each of whom has specialty training in geriatric mental health.

The outpatient clinic, located on the same floor, is staffed by a psychiatrist, a psychologist, a nurse specialist with a master's degree, a nurse specializing in the education and care of ECT patients and their families, a social worker expert in discharge planning for the inpatient unit, and an occupational therapist. The psychiatrist also functions as the program's medical director; the psychologist serves as the program coordinator. The nurse clinician works in the area of outreach, visiting nursing homes, agencies, and day-care programs to observe and define patient problems and recommend treatment alternatives. Team members provide evaluation of patients in the geriatric medicine clinic and provide consultation in the emergency room and general hospital. If possible, patients are brought to the geriatric psychiatry outpatient clinic for assessment and recommendations.

Private psychiatrists who admit their patients to the program are invited to become part of the team; they may utilize those portions of the program that are appropriate for the patient and his or her family. The private psychiatrist bills the patient for the time spent in assessment and treatment; the hospital-based team renders services to the patient for which the private psychiatrist is not qualified or is not reimbursed. Thus, this model provides the private practitioner with a system in which comprehensive, state-of-the-art geriatric psychiatric assessment and treatment is not compromised by limitations imposed by a solo or group private practice.

The teaching team (still being built) currently consists of geriatric medicine fellows from two different area medical schools and residents in either psychiatry or family medicine. Medical student rotation and a geriatric psychiatry fellowship program are in the planning phase.

Office-Based Psychogeriatric Practice

As mentioned in Chapter 2, 60% of most geriatric mental health services in this country are provided in the private sector. This model is an outgrowth of the historic, unsystematized, fee-for-service manner by which medicine has been organized in this country (Stein, in press). As such, there are multiple forces that shape the character of the private mental health care sector for geriatric patients. Geriatric patients seek care from private practitioners with varying degrees of satisfaction (Stein et al. 1989) and may access mental health care from different entry points, such as private offices, nursing home referrals, or inpatient units. Multiple entry points require psychiatrists to be flexible and able to treat patients in different settings at different points in time. Thus, the disposition, education, and personal inclination of private practitioners may have considerable influence on how private mental health services are delivered to geriatric patients (Stein, in press).

In recent years, the private health care system has also shaped the distribution and mix of mental health services provided for geriatric patients. From the per-spective of the private practitioner, these influences have been depicted as external restrictions, such as governmental regulation and legislation (fee structure regula-tion by the Health Care Financing Administration, or prescribing practices of psychotropic medication through the Omnibus Reconciliation Act of 1987, 1989, and 1990), insurance industry regulation (restrictions on mental health care ben-efits, precertification and continued stay criteria), peer review, malpractice litiga-tion, and physician and patient attitudes toward mental health (Klein et al. 1984; Ford and Sbordane 1980; Stein, in press). What is clear from present trends is that those clinicians who are private practitioners and who elect to treat geriatric patients will need skills that extend beyond an adequate scientific knowledge base of how to manage mental health problems in late life. They will also be required to develop a sophisticated, user-friendly practice environment that emphasizes effi-cient management practices, advocates for improved patient access for services, and remains responsive to ever-changing rules in the regulatory sector.

There are a variety of private practice models that can be used by private practitioners to serve as templates for private geriatric mental health services. Common to these models are special concerns that Stein (in press) suggests clinicians pay attention to when offering geriatric services:

1. Reasonable fee structure and billing procedures;
2. Patient accessibility to services;
3. Physician availability to see patients in nontraditional settings;
4. Flexible appointment scheduling;
5. Communicating clearly, quickly, and effectively with the patient and family or other concerned individual;
6. Expression of concern for the patient; and
7. Expression of confidence by the clinician that help *can* be given.

These features are commonsensibly put, but are often overlooked by practic-ing clinicians. A more detailed discussion of the mental health evaluation/assess-ment of the elderly patient is described by Goldstein (1990).

Psychiatrists who elect to treat geriatric patients must remember that for a large majority of these patients, the apprehension of seeing a psychiatrist for the first time in late life is overwhelming. The personal attributes of the physician and staff, the office or hospital environment, and the degree of medical professional-ism may be important factors in determining whether or not a patient participates in treatments that are offered.

Chapter 4

Department of Veterans Affairs Psychogeriatric Programs: Integrated Continuity of Care

The Veterans Administration was established in 1930 and renamed as the Department of Veterans Affairs (VA) in 1989. The Veterans Health Administration (VHA), the medical arm of the VA, supervises the largest organized health care system in the United States. Though the total number of veterans is anticipated to decrease from 28.6 million in 1980 to 17.1 million by 2020, veterans age 65 and over are anticipated to increase from 3.0 million (10.5% of total) in 1980 to 7.8 million (45.6% of total) by 2020 (Heltman and Adler 1990). Spanning the 50 states and Puerto Rico, are 159 VA medical centers (VAMC) including 13 two-division centers. These medical centers include 172 hospitals, 339 outpatient clinics, 126 VA nursing homes, and 32 domiciliaries. The VHA also provides partial federal support for an additional 162 community nursing homes, 55 state nursing homes, and 44 state veterans' domiciliaries (Department of Veterans Affairs 1990). Fully 125 of the 159 VA medical centers maintain formal affiliations with medical schools.

In fiscal year 1990, 12,145 full- and part-time physicians and many staff from other health care disciplines treated a total of 2,564,328 outpatients and more than 575,700 inpatients in VA facilities. The average daily bed census (ADC) across all facilities was 46,728. More than 191,400 patients were discharged from psychiatric services with an ADC of 14,526. The ADC of VA nursing homes was 11,787.

Recognizing the growing number of older veterans, the VHA began to establish designated psychogeriatric programs in the late 1970s.[1] More recently, the VA

---

[1] The term "psychogeriatric" was adopted to include geriatric psychiatry, geriatric medicine, geropsychology, and other disciplines that focus on treatment, training, and research involving elderly patients with significant mental, emotional, and/or behavioral problems, often in combination with medical problems.

Office of Strategic Planning has collaborated with the VA Mental Health and Behavioral Sciences Service and a number of working groups from field hospitals to develop a program that spans the full continuum of care for all VA psychiatric patients. The VA then adopted a policy requiring psychogeriatric programs to implement an integrated continuum of care matching the type of service to the level of care required by the patient (Department of Veterans Affairs 1991).

In addition, the VHA gradually has been expanding its primary emphasis from acute high-technology care to include geriatric and extended care services. Over the last 10 years, the VHA Geriatric and Extended Care Service has established 75 hospital-based home care teams, 5 pilot palliative care (hospice) units, 15 VA adult day health-care programs, 100 contract adult health care programs, 80 geriatric evaluation units (GEUs), and 15 Geriatric Research Education and Clinical Centers (GRECCs).

Psychogeriatric patients account for 2.4% of all VAMC admissions; however, such patients are responsible for almost 23% of total care days. In stark contrast to other loci of care for mentally ill elderly people, the VAMC's inpatient psychiatric population is 97% male. For example, women represent fully 65% of older patients in private psychiatric and private general hospitals and 60% of the population in public acute care facilities (Milazzo-Sayre et al. 1987). VAMCs serve only 7% of all psychiatric patients age 65 and over treated in inpatient units nationwide. Across all age groups, 35% of VAMC inpatient unit diagnoses are alcohol- or drug-related (Department of Veterans Affairs 1982).

Traditionally, much of the impetus for development of psychogeriatric programs has come from individual medical centers. In 1978, psychogeriatric programs were established at VAMCs in Salt Lake City, Utah; Palo Alto, California; Lyons, New Jersey; the Bronx, New York; Portland, Oregon; Salisbury, North Carolina; and San Antonio, Texas. The mutual interests in geriatric psychiatry in these programs led to national meetings on geriatric psychiatry in 1982 (Department of Veterans Affairs 1982). Recently, VAMCs have requested support for 12 new geriatric psychiatry programs, 8 new or expanded units, 2 psychiatric nursing home units, a psychogeriatric day treatment center, and a new clinic. The VA plans to develop 20 new Alzheimer's disease programs and 20 multilevel psychogeriatric programs within the next 6 years. At the same time, the VA Mental Health and Behavioral Sciences Service has responded to the need for additional numbers of well-trained psychogeriatricians by making funds available for eight fellowship sites in geriatric psychiatry.

A series of preliminary informal surveys of 50 selected VAMCs conducted in 1988 and 1990 sought to identify characteristics of psychogeriatric patients and to establish parameters for geriatric psychiatry programs. Unfortunately, no single set of characteristics for either patient or program achieved consensus. To resolve this dilemma, the VA created a VA Psychogeriatric Field Advisory Group to prepare a systemwide program inventory and a Psychogeriatric Program Guide. Because that material has not yet been developed, the Task Force received descriptions of examples of care in geriatric psychiatry programs in VA systems around the country. The programs are described in terms of their goals, modalities of services, staffing patterns, educational and research activities, and unique features that contribute to patient and/or family care.

Case Study: Geriatric Research, Education, and Clinical Center (GRECC; Minneapolis, Minnesota)

Mr. E., a 74-year-old World War II veteran, was referred by phone from the mental health clinic where he was being seen for persistent depression and possible memory loss. His condition had worsened since the death of a married daughter in an automobile accident. The medical clinic was also following Mr. E. for ongoing treatment of poorly controlled hypertension and chronic obstructive pulmonary disease. After speaking with Mr. and Mrs. E., the GRECC nurse mailed them an information packet describing the GRECC Memory Loss Clinic.

Mr. and Mrs. E. completed the intake form, providing answers to questions about the nature and extent of Mr. E.'s memory problems, depression, and medical history. When the form was returned, an appointment was scheduled for the E.s to visit the clinic. The new patient evaluation for Mr. E. consisted of a thorough history of his cognitive, affective, behavioral, and physical problems, coupled with a detailed physical and neurological examination. Daily living and safety issues were addressed, and financial and social resources were reviewed. The outpatient workup included blood studies, a computed tomography scan, and formal neuropsychological and functional examinations. After all studies were completed and reviewed, the GRECC staff held a family meeting with Mr. and Mrs. E. and their two daughters to review the evaluation, diagnosis, and prognosis and to outline recommendations and options for future care needs. A schedule was then set up to monitor the progression of the veteran's memory loss and the alleviation of his depression. Mrs. E. attended the caregiver education series at the GRECC and continues to contact GRECC staff, as needed, for advice regarding behavior changes and need for community support.

GRECCs were conceived by the VA in 1973 as a mechanism through which research, education, and clinical achievements in geriatrics and gerontology could be integrated. The Minneapolis GRECC is one of three with a specific focus on geriatric psychiatry. Training and education of a variety of health professionals is a major part of the program's mission. The affiliation with the University of

Minnesota School of Medicine involves training for medical residents, geriatric medicine fellows, geriatric psychiatry fellows, and residents from both services, as well as students in medicine, nursing, pharmacy, psychology, and social work. Regular geriatric psychiatry consultation to the nearby State Veterans Home and community nursing homes is part of the training/service program. The GRECC hosts both geriatric medicine and geriatric psychiatry fellowship programs. Fellows rotate through all of the GRECC's psychogeriatric programs and through the inpatient and outpatient psychiatry service as part of their training.

The majority of elderly patients seen in both inpatient and outpatient programs in this model present with complex multisystem medical and psychiatric problems requiring close collaboration among specialists. To meet their needs, the GRECC has a total of 45 beds, including 10 psychiatric beds and 35 intermediate medicine beds integrated within a medical/psychiatric-oriented ward. Patient length-of-stay is 2 to 3 weeks, during which time an extensive interdisciplinary evaluation of both patient and family is undertaken. A treatment plan is established and implemented, and a discharge plan is written. Program patients most often return to their referring physician in the hospital or community or move to long-term care facilities in the community or to the nearby VA long-term care medical center in St. Cloud. Another type of patient group admitted to the 10 dedicated psychiatric beds are those involved in a clinical or health-services research protocol under the direction of a GRECC staff member. These projects involve aspects of geriatric neuropsychiatry and may include patient and caregiver participation. Two respite beds also are available on the inpatient service as part of the family support program.

The overall GRECC clinical staff consists of two psychiatrists, an internist, a neurologist, three geriatric nurse-practitioners, one Ph.D. neuropsychologist, a psychometrician, a social worker, an occupational therapist, and nursing and support staff assigned to the larger 45-bed geriatric ward and clinics. Candidates for a geriatric pharmacology doctoral program and psychiatry and medical rehabilitation residents rotate through the program.

The GRECC provides a host of other programs and services as well. It maintains a weekly Dementia Clinic that provides interdisciplinary comprehensive evaluation, treatment, and follow-up for patients and families. A 36-bed ward located within the Extended Care Center (ECC) focuses on geriatric patients with combined medical/psychiatric problems who need long-term rehabilitation services. A geriatric psychiatrist is part of the interdisciplinary ward team. Similar consultation/liaison (C/L) services are provided to inpatient medicine, neurology, and psychiatric wards for geriatric patients exhibiting cognitive-behavioral problems. These beds are used for two types of geriatric patients: those referred from the GRECC outpatient clinic or other medical center clinics, and those referred from Admissions who are exhibiting unusual or inappropriate cognitive or behavior problems. In further C/L activity, the geriatric fellows also provide support for the ECC and Adult Day Health Care programs.

A unique Adapted Work Program (AWP) has been established and supports 12 outpatients diagnosed with early dementia. This program offers them employment in various departments of the hospital. Current jobs include making staff name plates, folding brochures, rolling bandages, and making salads. Patients are paid biweekly in cash from the hospital cashier from funds donated by volunteer organizations. Work is brought to them in a special area near the GRECC, and the level of work is adapted to their individual levels of cognitive capacity. Staff working with these patients include a geriatric nurse-practitioner, an occupational therapist, and a certified occupational therapy assistant. A pretest and 18-month follow-up study of the AWP patients revealed that the patients' level of depression had decreased based on findings from both the Geriatric Depression Scale (GDS; Yesavage et al. 1983) and a clinical examination.

Moreover, a newly formed Geriatric Psychiatry Clinic has been developed as part of the mental health clinic in the psychiatry service. It operates 1 day a week and is staffed by two geriatric psychiatrists, a geriatric medicine nurse-practitioner, and a social worker. Elderly patients, generally with both psychiatric and chronic medical problems, are assessed, treated, and followed by this clinic in an attempt to provide a semblance of integrated medicine, psychiatry, and primary care.

Case Study: VAMC Geriatric Psychiatry Program (West Los Angeles, California)

Mr. F., a 65-year-old veteran with a history of hypertension, was otherwise well until an acute onset of right-sided weakness and speaking difficulty. He was admitted to the VAMC and a left cerebrovascular accident (CVA) was diagnosed. Although the right-sided weakness improved with rehabilitative therapy, Mr. F. developed symptoms of major depression and became suicidal. Once medically stable, he was transferred to the Psychogeriatric Inpatient Unit, where he responded well to nortriptyline and psychotherapy.

Mr. F. was discharged to his home, followed by the Geriatric Outpatient Clinic, and maintained on medication. However, when Mrs. F. died suddenly, Mr. F. became isolated and substantially more depressed. His outpatient geriatric psychiatrist referred him to the Geriatric Day Treatment Program. The group activities helped mitigate his loneliness and depression, and he was able to remain in the community for another year. Mr. F. subsequently had another CVA and could no longer care for himself. He was admitted to the Nursing Home Care Unit, where he remains today.

The mission of the Geriatric Psychiatry Program is to provide the highest quality care to aged veterans with psychiatric disorders. Optimum care requires a continuum of resources, including inpatient, outpatient, consultation, day-care, and nursing home programs, as well as multidisciplinary services that include psychiatry, behavioral neurology, nursing, social work, psychology, rehabilitation medicine, medical-surgical consultation, and physical and occupational therapy. Optimum care also demands the availability of evaluative techniques, including laboratory, neuroimaging, and neuropsychological approaches.

The program's inpatient unit staffing levels are as follows: 2.5 psychiatrists, 3 registered nurses, 2 licensed practical nurses, 3 nurses' aides, 1 half-time psychologist, 1.5 social workers, and 1 clerk. They service a unit of 39 beds; patients have an average length of stay of 28 days on the unit.

A geriatric day treatment unit, serving 30 patients, is staffed by a physician, a social worker, a registered nurse, a social services worker, a recreational therapist, and a nutritionist.

The outpatient clinic is staffed part-time by a psychiatrist, a psychologist, a social worker, and a registered nurse with expertise in geriatrics and mental health. Up to 300 visits are made to the clinic annually.

A nursing home care unit (now serving 60 residents, but soon to be expanded to meet the needs of 100) is staffed by a physician and part-time social workers, rehabilitation therapists, and psychologists.

Two specialized programs are also operating under the aegis of the Geriatric Psychiatry Program: a Dementia/Neurobehavior Clinic, with approximately 500 visits per year and a 15-bed (average 24-day stay) neurobehavioral inpatient unit. Together, these services are staffed at the levels of 1.25 physicians, 1.75 registered nurses, 1 half-time occupational therapist, .75 social worker, and 1 clerk.

The activities of the Program extend beyond clinical care into professional training, providing hands-on training for two geriatric psychiatry fellows, a neurobehavior fellow, a geriatric medicine fellow, and a general psychiatry resident.

VAMC Geriatric Psychiatry Program (Miami, Florida)

This multi-institutional program in geriatric psychiatry, involved in clinical care, research, and professional training, maintains a close working relationship with the University of Miami, Highland Park Psychiatric Pavilion, Mount Sinai Medical Center, and other community institutions. These intermeshed relationships help the facility maintain professional interest and attract high-quality psychiatrists and other health care professionals to the psychogeriatrics program.

Because of the complex comorbidities seen in elderly patients, the geriatric psychiatry program both collaborates and integrates with the geriatric medicine program. Such an interdisciplinary approach for the evaluation and care of both patient and family is an essential component of the program. Equally important is the concept of a continuum of care, ranging from acute care to medically supported independent community living.

The integrated psychogeriatric care within the VA medical center includes a variety of facilities. A 25-bed acute psychiatry ward is staffed for both general psychiatric patients and geriatric psychiatry patients by 1 psychiatrist, 1 social worker, 1 head nurse, 5 registered nurses, 2 licensed practical nurses, and 6 nursing assistants. A psychiatric consultation/liaison service, composed of a psychiatrist and three psychiatric fellows, responds to requests from inpatient medicine, surgery, neurology, and rehabilitation medicine. A 60-bed nursing home unit is staffed by 7.5 full-time equivalent physicians, 1 head nurse, 12 registered nurses, two licensed practical nurses, 13 nursing assistants, 1 nurse-practitioner, 1 half-time psychologist, 1 social worker, and 1 quarter-time recreational therapist. A 10-bed geriatric evaluation and management unit (GEM) is housed within the nursing home care unit. Patients in that unit are given an extensive interdisciplinary evaluation before placement.

Several other programs are of particular relevance for the psychogeriatric patient. A 20-bed unit within the nursing home care program specializes in the care of dementia patients whose length of stay is anticipated to be at least 6 months. A thorough interdisciplinary evaluation and treatment program are afforded all patients placed in this unit, the goal of which is to permit community placement. The dementia program is located within a 60-bed locked unit on the fourth floor of the nursing home care facility. Plans are under way for the division of the unit to ensure separate care facilities for patients with dementia and those with other psychiatric disorders. Respite care is also available through the nursing home care unit. Up to 10 beds can be made available for patients requiring 1 to 2 weeks of care to relieve caregivers. Finally, the facility maintains a geriatric outpatient clinic that focuses on the geriatric psychiatry patient 1 day a week. It provides an extensive multidisciplinary examination and treatment for patients referred either from the medical center or from the community. The clinic is staffed by a supervised psychiatric fellow, a nurse-practitioner, and a social worker. Up to 200 visits per year have been logged by the psychogeriatric clinic.

With close working relationships with local public and private facilities and with the University of Miami Medical School, the VAMC has been able to undertake a variety of geriatric psychiatry training and research activities. In collaboration with the Medical School, the VAMC has developed fellowship programs in both geriatric medicine and geriatric psychiatry. These programs provide comprehensive training across multiple clinical service sites, include intensive supervised research training, and permit significant teaching opportunities. Moreover, a number of specific research commitments span the VAMC-University of Miami Medical School relationship. Ongoing research activities span basic, clinical, and epidemiologic study and include investigation into areas such as psychiatric evaluation in nursing home settings, epilepsy and aging, effectiveness and cost of adult day care, hypertension in geriatric patients, lateralized brain impairment, new drug trials for the treatment of dementia, neuropsychological evaluation in Alzheimer's disease and other dementias, caregiver burden, comparative studies across older ethnic populations, biochemical and immunological changes in late life and in patients with dementia, autonomic reactivity and learning in Alzheimer's disease, the role of the serotonergic system in Alzheimer's dementia-depression complex, and gender and longevity.

Sources of Support

The Department of Veterans Affairs cares for the needs of some 27 million veterans with an annual budget of approximately $30 billion. As with other items in the federal budget, the amount appropriated to the VA each year is negotiated between the President and Congress, reflecting compromises among a myriad of political and economic factors. Approximately $12 billion of the $30 billion budget is directed toward medical care provided in 172 hospitals, 339 outpatient clinics, 126 nursing homes, and 32 domiciliaries. In addition, the VA medical budget helps support selected state nursing and veterans homes and contracts with military facilities, selected non-VA medical centers, clinics, and clinicians located in areas far from VA facilities. Eligibility for VA care is established by law and generally focuses on veterans requiring medical care as the result of injury or disease related to active duty in the military and for veterans who are essentially medically indigent.

In 1990, approximately $1.2 billion was directed toward a wide range of mental health needs for eligible veterans, including those needs resulting from homelessness, substance abuse, posttraumatic stress disorder, chronic mental illness, and aging. Funds are divided among clinical facilities annually by the VA Central Office in Washington, using a complex allocation process that reflects historical factors, anticipated needs, and centrally directed priorities. Although policies, management, and overall facility budgets emanate from the VA Central Office, each individual facility director has considerable autonomy regarding the use of funds at that particular facility. Because there is no VA funding category specific to geriatric psychiatry, the proportion of funds spent on geriatric psychiatry, locally or nationally, is not discernible. Although most facilities address the mental health needs of elderly veterans through existing programs in psychiatry, medicine, geriatrics, or extended care, there is currently little emphasis on or visibility for geriatric psychiatry per se.

The low priority given to developing an organized, comprehensive focus on psychogeriatric issues by the VA nationally, or by its medical school affiliates, stands in distinct contrast to the challenge posed by aging veterans. Indeed, this gap has led some VA clinicians to request more funds to educate new professionals in the principles of geriatric psychiatry, to integrate psychogeriatric knowledge into existing programs, and to create new programs where demand and clinical interest are evident.

Chapter 5

APA Professional Activities and Biographical Directory Survey—Focus on Geriatric Psychiatry

Reporting on models of practice in geriatric psychiatry and their availability, accessibility, and affordability for the elderly needs to go hand in hand with a review of training, teaching, research, and service activities of the psychiatrists who have made themselves available for the practice of geriatric psychiatry. Although we are aware of the unique training and service needs for the mental health of the elderly and their caregivers, the absence of specialty status (added qualifications or equivalency) in geriatric psychiatry during the 1982 and 1988 American Psychiatric Association surveys limits differentiation of specialized service provisions for the elderly from that of general psychiatry. However, as "research questions" have been added to the surveys since 1982, cumulative data are emerging gradually in the geriatric psychiatry arena. The APA has published nine biographical directories of its members since 1941. For the 1988 survey, special topics were proposed by APA member components and by APA staff. Questions about patient characteristics by demographics and diagnosis, psychiatrists' special interests, customary services, worksettings, and economics of their practice were included.

Whereas the 1982 survey listed Geriatrics/Gerontology as "nonpsychiatric postgraduate training" and Geriatric Psychiatry as a "special interest," the 1988 survey listed Fellowships in Geriatric Psychiatry under training and included nursing homes as one of the worksettings. The two surveys differ in other substantive ways. In 1982, all surveys included questions regarding the age range of patients treated; in 1988 only a randomly selected sample of 20% surveyed included these questions. In 1982, the total number of psychiatrists for whom data were analyzed was 19,735, which represented a response rate of 64.4%. In 1988, data of 19,948 were analyzed, which represented a response rate of 67.7%. It is, of course, understood that there are differences between survey respondents and nonrespondents. However, because of the size of the sample, it is considered unlikely that this has created large distortions in the data (Koran 1987). Because the response rate was high and consistent in both surveys and the 1988 subsample was randomly selected, it is permissible to make inferences from comparisons of the results of these two surveys (J. Lyons, personal communication, January 1992).

Though aware of the above limitations, the Task Force set out to formulate profiles of psychiatrists who participated in the two surveys and who identified themselves as seeing in their practices 1) less than 20% patients age 65 and over, 2) 20% or more patients age 65 and over, and 3) primarily patients age 65 and over, defined as 50% or more. The group who saw 20% or more elderly (defined as age 65 and over) constituted 7.3% of all respondents in 1982 and 11% in 1988, a statistically significant difference ($\chi^2 = 31.6$, df = 1, $P < .0001$). The group who saw more than 50% elderly constituted 1.8% in the 1982 and 2.3% in the 1988 survey, indicating an upward trend in an altogether very small group of 84 in 1988, 27.4% of whom were foreign trained and reported their worksettings to be in state hospitals.

Subsequently, a profile of age, gender, race, place of medical education, and primary worksetting was established for psychiatrists with 20% or more and 20% or less elderly in their patient population. This profile revealed the following.

Age

In 1982, psychiatrists under 50 years of age were less likely than those age 50 and over to be in the practice category of having more than 20% elderly patients. This difference was no longer significant in 1988, which can partly be accounted for by the increased proportion of younger psychiatrists among the respondents.

Gender

In both surveys, men respondents were slightly more likely than women respondents to have a 20% or more geriatric caseload, in spite of the fact that the overall proportion of women respondents rose from 1982 to 1988. The gender differences between psychiatrists with a caseload of more than 20% elderly patients in the 1988 survey is outlined in Table 3.

Race/Ethnicity

Psychiatrists of color were more likely to have a caseload of 20% or more of geriatric patients in 1982 than did Caucasian psychiatrists. Their representation

Table 3. 1988 survey: gender differences of psychiatrists with a greater than 20% geriatric caseload

Gender	Total N	$N > 20\%$	%
Male	3,125	363	11.6
Female	714	63	8.5

$\chi^2 = 5.17$, df = 1, $P < .03$.

amongst those with this volume of geriatric patients diminished slightly in 1988.

The proportion of elderly served across psychiatrists with different ethnic backgrounds in the 1988 survey was provocative, though in view of the relatively small numbers of respondents in some ethnic groups, no conclusions can be drawn. The overwhelming majority of respondents were Caucasian; therefore, statistical comparisons could be misleading. All 5 responding American Indian psychiatrists in 1988 reported serving 20% or more geriatric caseloads. There were no differences between African American and Hispanic/Latino psychiatrists and Caucasian psychiatrists. However, amongst Asian or Pacific Islander psychiatrists, a significantly higher proportion served 20% or more geriatric patients than did Caucasian psychiatrists ($P < .03$). Response bias should be taken into account, because there was substantial variation among racial/ethnic categories in response rate to the member survey. Whereas Caucasian APA members responded at a rate of 76.3%, those of Asian/Pacific Island heritage responded at a rate of 65.7%, black/African Americans at 55.2%, and Hispanic/Latino at 29.3%.

Place of Medical Education

In 1982, foreign-trained psychiatrists were significantly overrepresented among those with a volume of over 20% geriatric caseloads. Though this difference was no longer significant in 1988, it remained significant among psychiatrists with a caseload of more than 50% elderly patients. This can most likely be attributed to the fact that a high proportion of state hospital patients have aged and many foreign-trained graduates are employed in state hospitals (T. Dial, personal communication, January 1992).

Work Setting

In both the 1982 and 1988 surveys, psychiatrists in private practice settings, community mental health centers, and health maintenance organizations (HMOs) were much less likely to have a caseload of 20% elderly patients than those with primary worksettings in hospital environments, whether academic, private, government, or otherwise. The decline between 1982 and 1988 is also a reflection of the overall decline in the number of psychiatrists in private practice. We were unable to determine the number of psychiatrists whose primary worksetting was the Veterans Health Administration because this group was merged with psychiatrists reporting their primary worksetting to be in federal hospitals and the military.

Other interesting characteristics emerged when *special interests* and *customary services* rendered by the group of psychiatrists with at least 20% of their patients in the geriatric category were analyzed. The list of about 50 different special interests included a mixture of types of disorders, types of treatments, sites of practice, and types of work. Approximately 50% indicated a special interest in each of the following: geriatric psychiatry; affective, anxiety, organic, and schizophrenic disorders; psychopharmacology; consultation/liaison; and inpatient and outpatient psychiatry. A lower percentage chose the remaining as special interests, with only 6.6% indicating interest in women's issues in spite of the high percentage of women patients and women caregivers in the geriatric population. It should be noted that the question in the survey was "women/feminist." We might speculate and hope that had the question been worded "women/aging and/or women/caregiving" that we might have found a closer relationship between this special interest and the number of psychiatrists with a caseload of 20% or more elderly patients. Selected special interests that were reported by a statistically significant higher number of psychiatrists with 20% or more caseload of elderly when compared with psychiatrists who did not are listed in Table 4. The total number of respondents in this subsample who identified themselves as having less than 20% elderly patients in their caseload was 2,940, and the total of those with more than 20% elderly patients in their caseload was 396 (only APA members were included).

As a treatment modality, psychopharmacology ranked high as a special interest of psychiatrists with a 20% elderly patient caseload, whereas family/couple problems and psychoanalysis ranked low.

Of the list of customary services, those performed by a statistically significant higher percentage of psychiatrists with a 20% elderly patient caseload are reflected in Table 5. Their total number was 383, whereas the total number of psychiatrists with less than 20% elderly patients in their caseload who responded to this part of the questionnaire was 3,073 (APA members and nonmembers were included).

In addition, it is of interest to note that psychiatrists with at least 20% of their patient population age 65 and over practiced individual therapy in conjunction with chemotherapy with statistically significant greater frequency than their colleagues with fewer elderly patients in their practice. The latter practiced individual therapy without chemotherapy with statistically significant greater frequency. Though small in total number ($N = 30$; 0.8%), as mentioned previously, the 1988 survey included a group that had had a fellowship in geriatric psychiatry. Of

Table 4. 1988 survey: special interests

Special interest	> 20% Elderly Total N = 396 N	%	< 20% Elderly Total N = 2,940 N	%	χ^2 (df = 1)
Geriatric psychiatry	243	59.1	747	25.4	195.4***
Neurology/neuropsychiatry	92	22.4	389	13.2	58.4***
Administrative psychiatry	119	29	707	24.1	4.4*
Consultation/liaison	208	50.6	914	32.2	60.9***
Emergency psychiatry	115	28	615	20.9	10.2***
Inpatient psychiatry	196	47.9	1,183	40.3	8.0**
Organic mental disorders	170	41.4	624	21.2	79.8***
Affective disorders	269	65.5	1,737	59.1	5.9*
Chronic pain management	89	21.7	368	12.5	24.8***
Somatoform/psychophysical	95	23.1	507	17.3	8.1**
Psychopharmacology	249	60.6	1,499	51	13.0***
Family/couple problems	106	25.8	1,027	35	13.0***
Psychoanalysis	32	7.8	589	20	35.0***

*$P < .05.$ **$P < .01.$ ***$P < .001.$

Table 5. 1988 survey: customary services

Customary service	> 20% Elderly Total N = 383 N	%	< 20% Elderly Total N = 3,073 N	%	χ^2 (df = 1)
Diagnostic assessment	282	73.6	2,105	68.5	4.0*
Laboratory tests	71	18.5	439	14.3	4.6*
Nonpsychiatric MD consult	239	62.4	1,517	49.4	22.6***
Electroconvulsive therapy	99	25.8	296	9.6	86.9***
Psychopharmacotherapy	302	78.9	2,104	68.5	16.9***
Forensic/legal consult	104	27.2	648	21.1	7.0**
Inpatient treatment	200	52.2	1,391	45.3	6.4*
Nursing home consult	110	28.7	305	9.9	112.1***

*$P < .05.$ **$P < .01.$ ***$P < .001.$

the 30 psychiatrists with geriatric psychiatry fellowships, only 11 (36.7%) had a high volume (20%) geriatric practice; but the average proportion of geriatric cases was significantly higher among this group when compared with all other psychiatrists. One reason for this finding could be that the amount of time spent in research is nearly three times as much for the psychiatrists with geriatric fellowships.

In these survey data, it is not as yet clear what constitutes a geriatric psychiatrist and what constitutes a psychiatrist who sees elderly patients. As geriatric psychiatry advances, survey data can be obtained in such a way that it will reflect not only how many elderly patients a psychiatrist sees. Future surveys will be able to determine personal interest, specialty training, certification, and more varied modalities and sites of treatment where elderly patients and their families and caregivers could or ought to be the recipients of medical mental health care and the effect this has on psychiatrists' expenditure of time, income, and professional satisfaction. Future content and analysis of survey questionnaires can include the special sites, conditions, and treatments that focus on the needs the elderly and their families and caregivers have for medical mental health care. These surveys have the potential of revealing where psychiatrists are needed, what changes have occurred over time, and how policy-making should be influenced by the trends discovered.

Many questions remain to be answered. Do psychiatrists with a high volume of elderly patients have lower income and work longer hours? Is there a shortage of psychiatrists willing to see the elderly, their families, and other caregivers? Is there a reluctance on the part of the elderly to see psychiatrists? Is there a reluctance on the part of primary care physicians, internists, surgeons, gerontologists, other physicians, and nonmedical mental health workers to refer elderly patients and their families to psychiatrists? How can these disparities be remedied? Do medical students and residents lack training in geriatric psychiatry? Are there too few fellows in geriatric psychiatry to become the future teachers, researchers, and practitioners in issues related to the mental health of our aging population?

Future APA surveys have the potential of advancing our knowledge in these domains.

Chapter 6

A Canadian Model of Comprehensive Geriatric Psychiatry Care

The difficulty in developing comprehensive programs is reflected in their scarcity in the overall mental health service network for the elderly. The model that follows is an example of one approach to the translation of theoretical principles into a working system.

Background

The anticipation of a new geriatric hospital on the campus of Baycrest Center, Toronto, Ontario, several years ago stimulated the concept of a planned department of psychiatry capable of serving both the patients and residents of the institution as well as various community needs. From 1955 to 1980, psychiatric service was limited to intermittent, occasional consultation service to residents, provided on an ad hoc basis. No community psychiatric services existed. Although limited in scope, the clinical excellence of the psychiatric consultation helped stimulate an awareness of the larger complex psychiatric needs of the patients in the institution. The new plans for an expanded department, in turn, stimulated the development of community-oriented services and spearheaded the development of medical outreach in a variety of programs. The Center's administration, while initially cautious, soon embraced the concept of a comprehensive psychiatry program, and, in 1980, it incorporated the plans into an application for government funding. Indeed, the unique nature of the psychiatry plan became one strong impetus for the government to grant special status to Baycrest in allocating funds in excess of that usually given to chronic care facilities.

Facility Philosophy and Services

The Baycrest Center has been developed based on a philosophy of a continuum of care for geriatric patients. The Department of Psychiatry at Baycrest shares that philosophy, serving not only patients and residents of the institution but also various needs of community-dwelling elderly patients. Thus, the Department of Psychiatry primarily conducts and supports active care programs. It maintains an academic program that provides training to residents in general psychiatry and fellows in geriatric psychiatry seeking specialized training, as well as other disciplines on the health-care team. Integrated into the service and training components is an active research program, currently focused on clinical efficacy trials and competency evaluation.

The basic funding for the Department of Psychiatry comes from the "global" budget for the institution that is provided by the Ministry of Health's Institutional Branch (Table 6).

This budget funds nonmedical staff needed to provide support for an inpatient unit, a day hospital, parts of a consultation/liaison (C/L) team, and outpatient services. All psychiatrists are paid primarily through direct fee-for-service for patient care, which is reimbursed through the universal medical insurance plan (Ontario Hospital Insurance Plan [OHIP]). However, indirect services, such as meetings, teaching, conferences, and so on, which occupy up to 50% of the psychiatrist's time, are not supported through OHIP. To pay for some of the nonfunded activities, the Ministry of Health provides an additional grant (sessional fees) to the Baycrest department to offset nonremunerated administrative, clinical, and teaching time. The outpatient community programs are funded on special grants from the Community Mental Health Division of the Ministry of Health. These grants are made based on competitive special application that must go through a complex process of priority setting before funding is granted.

All patient-related activities are supported; there are no deductibles, no

---

Table 6. Baycrest Center for Geriatric Care—funding sources

Global institutional budget (provincial government)
Universal Health Insurance (OHIP)
Ministry of Health (Community Mental Health Branch)
  —special program funding
  —sessional grants
Private donations (Baycrest Foundation)
External research grants

copayments (except for private or semiprivate inpatient room charges), no uninsured patients, no regional insurance variations, and no financial limitations on services rendered. Thus, for example, the C/L service can focus with equal emphasis on patient, staff, and family intervention and do so for an extended period of time in the program's long-term care settings.

The Baycrest Center's programs span community-based and institution-based programs. The following community services are provided: day care, day social programs, special day programs for elderly patients with dementia, and an outreach program for burdened caregivers. Three separate facility-based settings are available for patients requiring admission, depending largely on patient preferences and needs.

The Terrace. An apartment building of approximately 250 beds, The Terrace provides central services, some shopping facilities, a full-time nursing clinic, a social work department, medical care provided by part-time physicians, and one meal per day. Residents of this facility must retain basic capacity for self-care, including the preparation of meals not otherwise provided and the arrangement of social and other activities.

The Jewish Home for the Aged (JHA). JHA is a 300-bed nursing facility with multiple levels of care. Twenty percent of the beds are devoted to special care for the cognitively impaired elderly. Another 20% are devoted to physically ill patients who require a high degree of nursing care. The balance of the beds are reserved for those elderly who cannot function independently but who maintain a degree of relative interpersonal stability and capacity for basic activities of daily living (ADL). The average age of JHA residents is approximately 84 years.

Baycrest Hospital. The third of the program's facilities, this 300-bed facility is devoted exclusively to geriatric care in both acute and chronic forms. Two-thirds (200) of the beds are occupied by long-stay patients, including those requiring either rehabilitative care or palliative care. Medical services are provided by family practitioners hired by the institution. Full-time medical nursing care is provided. The remaining 100 beds are reserved for acute care divided among various medical services including psychiatry, behavioral neurology, medical assessment, and rehabilitation. Although the acute care components of the hospital admit patients directly from the community, they do not serve as a point of entry to the chronic care components of Baycrest. Almost all acute admissions from the community are discharged to their home or to another appropriate facility. The hospital has full support services of all relevant medical specialties on a regular scheduled consulting basis. Complete up-to-date laboratory, radiology (excluding therapeutic radiation), physiotherapy, social work, audiology, speech, and pharmacy services are housed within the institution. Other services (such as high-technology scanning) are available through a formal relationship with a teaching general hospital.

Baycrest's Department of Psychiatry

The psychiatry department is but one component of the comprehensive services of the Center. Within this setting, the Department of Psychiatry, occupying nearly a full floor of the Baycrest Hospital, maintains five divisions, each with a program coordinator responsible for clinical, research, and educational activity within a given area. The divisions include an inpatient division, an outpatient division, a C/L division, a day hospital division, a competency clinic, and a community outreach team. Continuity of care is defined to encompass the full spectrum of treatment modalities from which to choose when determining need and level of care.

Under this system, access to care is no longer a problem for the patient. Although no emergency room service is provided for patients from the community, the Department of Psychiatry provides 24-hour service through a rotating on-call schedule. In this way, the Department is able to respond to emergencies arising in any patient registered in the Department's programs, or in any non-psychiatric patient elsewhere in the Center who experiences a psychiatric emergency.

The psychiatry staff positions number 13; of these, 7 are full-time in the facility. The remaining psychiatrists are hired on a part-time basis to provide specialized teaching or clinical services. Within this group is a specialized group therapist (8 hours/week) who coordinates the group therapy, teaching, and clinical activity; a family therapist (3 hours/week) who provides family therapy supervision and seminar teaching; a geriatric psychiatrist/psychoanalyst (8 hours/week) who is one of the psychotherapy supervisors; and other part-time clinical staff (approximately 15 hours/week) who are part of the outpatient follow-up and C/L services.

The 20-bed inpatient unit in the Department of Psychiatry maintains a nurse-patient ratio of 1:5 (days), 1:6.3 (evenings), and 1:10 (nights). One social worker is on staff. The unit also includes 1.5 occupational therapists and a half-time internist who provides both medical consultation and direct care. Electroconvulsive therapy (ECT) and anesthetic services are provided through liaison with one of the general hospitals in Toronto. Referrals to the inpatient unit are made by physicians in the community, other Baycrest Center programs, or other hospitals in the area.

Many of the patients referred to the inpatient unit have complex physical as well as emotional difficulties. A significant subgroup of patients admitted to Baycrest are Holocaust survivors who require additional expertise and sensitivity from staff members.

Patients and facility professionals share the understanding that admission to any part of the Center means that the Center will remain the caretaker. Occasionally, patients admitted from Baycrest Terrace to the inpatient unit for treatment of psychiatric disorders are not considered appropriate for return to Baycrest Terrace. In Canada, as in the United States, with the rising number of elderly, the treatment bottleneck often occurs at the time of admission to the nursing home. Patients unable to return to Baycrest Terrace are thus permitted to remain on the unit for up to 1 year or more while awaiting a JHA bed. Thus, for the most part, the continuity of care is institutional rather than personal. The personal level is reached when the community outreach team case managers "shadow" a patient's transit through the entire system.

The average length of stay is 93 days (much less for the active care group). In addition to the general complexity of the problems of patients presenting to the hospital for treatment, there are other significant problems contributing to the high length of stay—those with dementing illnesses and accompanying medical or behavioral problems, those with medical illness precluding nursing home admission (e.g., need for oxygen), or those with psychiatric illnesses for whom nursing homes are unable or unwilling to provide care. Such patients require careful and lengthy discharge arrangements. Usually a guarantee of readmission, a "money back guarantee" is required to facilitate the discharge. In the past, 20% of patients on the unit at any given time were inactive, awaiting discharge to appropriate settings. (Indeed, one patient remained nearly 3 years.) However, in the past year, admission and discharge criteria have been tightened to restrict admission to active cases. The costs of all care, regardless of length of stay, are covered fully by universal health insurance.

The outpatient service includes a geriatric psychiatry community team that evaluates and treats older patients referred by social service agencies to the assessment team. To the extent possible, the team refers patients for inpatient care only when deemed absolutely necessary. Under most circumstances, patients are linked to community-based outpatient services, whether provided by Baycrest or other entities. Selected patients may continue in active treatment provided by team members; others, also identified by the community team's assessment, may receive direct outpatient follow-up care from Baycrest staff psychiatrists. However, because of the limited number of staff psychiatrists, this aspect of the program remains unable to meet the full demand for services.

The day hospital program provides comprehensive assessment and treatment for 20–25 depressed patients over age 55 who need intensive daily psychiatric treatment, but who may continue to reside in the community. It is intended neither as a custodial nor placement alternative and has an average length of stay of 12 weeks. Staff include a psychiatrist, an in-house geriatrician, two nurses, an occupational therapist, and a social worker. A wide variety of group programs focus on the development and facilitation of life skills, practical skills of routine ADL, and use of recreational and supportive services in the community.

The C/L service has two major objectives: provision of psychiatric assessment and/or treatment to all identified patients and residents of Baycrest, and provision of staff support and education about psychiatric and behavioral problems. The Service includes two full-time psychiatrists, one full-time equivalent (FTE) psychiatric resident, two FTE nurse clinicians, and a part-time psychologist. As many as 5 new referrals to the service are made each week; an average of 34 visits for assessment, treatment, or follow-up are made weekly. The care model is based on a biopsychosocial approach, offering both elective and emergency consultations for patients and residents of the institution.

A competency clinic was established to provide clinical assessments and recommendations regarding judgments of competency and the necessity for guardianship of elderly patients. Staffed by a psychiatrist, a bioethicist, and a lawyer, the clinic provides clinical assessment and consultation regarding patient competency, undertakes research in competency-related areas of law, ethics, and psychiatry, and trains members of the Baycrest medical and support teams.

Although it receives extensive support from the government, Baycrest Center nonetheless remains an independently affiliated university institution. Students and residents of many disciplines train at Baycrest: medicine, psychiatry, neurology, psychology, nursing, and social work. The majority of teaching staff are full-time members of the Baycrest staff, with offices in the institution and virtually all their time devoted to Baycrest. Indeed, the Department of Psychiatry places substantial emphasis on education, as the largest of six teaching units in the division of geriatric psychiatry at the University of Toronto. Structured rounds, clinical and research conferences, and meetings provide both education and supervised experience for residents and fellows in the program. Two full-time residents in geriatric psychiatry are assigned to Baycrest for 6–12 months. Junior residents spend the majority of time on the inpatient service; more senior residents experience a combined C/L-outpatient rotation. In addition, the department has supported anywhere from one to three geriatric psychiatry fellows annually. Fellows are expected to undertake formal research activity, as well as to develop specialized clinical skills in geriatric psychiatry.

In this specialized model with its continuity of care, patient and family expectations are raised. Limits of program mandates must be well-defined and publicized clearly to eliminate the illusion that such a system can be all things to everyone. Although each service in itself can be considered a model of care, the unique nature of this program is its accessibility and its integrated approach to a range of patient care needs over time.

Chapter 7

International Perspectives on Psychogeriatric Models

Interest in the mental health concerns of our world's ever-aging population originated in the welfare societies of Northern Europe more than 30 years ago. At that time, many policymakers began to realize that the public health consequences of an aging population affect the entire population. Increased survival is accompanied by rising chronic disease—including increased incidence and prevalence of psychiatric disorders. The World Health Organization (WHO) began grappling with the area of mental illness in the elderly in 1958, publishing a series of technical reports on the subject in 1959, 1972, 1979, and 1985. The purpose of these reports was to highlight recent developments in psychogeriatric knowledge, to make recommendations on the outstanding needs for further research, to analyze the effectiveness of services, to promote international collaborations, and to disseminate that information to the 130 member nations of WHO. Already, in 1972, the WHO scientific psychogeriatric group advised that increased attention should be paid to the community caregivers who support mentally frail elderly people. This could better ensure continuity of care within the community, in lieu of unnecessary use of institutionalization. Implementation of these recommendations, unfortunately, has been the exception rather than the rule in many of the 130 WHO member nations.

As part of a WHO Health For All (HFA) planning initiative, researchers at the Johns Hopkins School of Hygiene and Public Health have developed a Computer Assisted Planning (CAP) software package that enables the organization to promote long-term health planning for the elderly through the year 2000 in each of the WHO member nations. CAP was adopted by the Canadian province of Manitoba and by Norway for actual planning purposes.

HFA planning for the year 2000 hopes to increase the average number of years that people will live free from major disease and disability by 10%. It also hopes to develop a common language to describe illness across nations. As part of that

53

effort, the Alcohol, Drug Abuse and Mental Health Administration (ADAMHA) joined with WHO in 1979 to codify a common nomenclature. The *Diagnostic and Statistical Manual of Mental Disorders, 4th Edition* and the *International Classification of Disease, 10th Edition*, both now under development, represent a coordinated classification effort. Through such collaboration, researchers will be better able to conduct cross-national epidemiologic studies to identify the actual prevalence and incidence of disorder and not differences in diagnostic practice.[1]

Interest in geriatric psychiatry and the need for diagnostic categories of psychopathology of late life and specialized psychiatric care for the elderly have been evidenced abroad for considerably greater time than in the United States. Models of care have been developed and tested more rigorously in Europe and Israel than in this country. To begin to examine such models, the Task Force initiated communications with 20 active foreign members of the International Psychogeriatric Association. The responses provide much of the material presented in this section of our report.

Although in no way intended to provide a thorough overview of the state of psychogeriatric care abroad, this chapter provides further fuel for the long-term care debate. For detailed information on activities in geriatric psychiatry in particular countries, the reader is referred to the section on International Psychogeriatric Developments in the *Journal of the International Psychogeriatric Association*.

Great Britain

Researchers and health services agencies in Great Britain have undertaken regional surveys and reports identifying the needs, services, training, and opportunities for geriatricians and psychogeriatricians on a regular basis over the past four decades (Arie 1986; Arie and Jolley 1982; Copeland 1984; Hemsi 1982; Kay et al. 1966; Norman 1980; Royal College of Physicians and Royal College of Psychiatrists 1989; Royal College of Psychiatrists/British Geriatric Society 1979; Wattis et al. 1981). Indeed, the theory underlying the concept of care models originated in the 1950s in Great Britain. It specified a number of ideals for model geriatric programs:

---

[1]One of the significant problems that arose in the London–New York portion of a larger United States–Great Britain cross-national project was the failure to correct for incompatible nomenclature in the two study sites. The epidemiological findings produced more information regarding differing nomenclature than they did regarding the relative incidence and prevalence of specific mental disorders (Copeland and Gurland 1985).

✦ Services should be designed to encourage maintenance of patients in their own homes, including the use of home assessment and day hospitals.

✦ Hospital treatment should be rapidly responsive and highly effective.

✦ Programs should emphasize the prevention of chronic disability.

✦ The quality of life in long-stay institutions should be improved.

✦ Programs should be attentive to the needs of caregivers and to mental health care providers.

Four models of care in Great Britain—in South Hampton, West Cornwall, Gloucestershire, and Goodmayes Hospital in London—that have adhered to these precepts were reviewed in the 1977 report of the American Psychiatric Association/National Mental Health Association's Joint Information Service (Glasscote et al. 1977).

Over time, these precepts have been translated into norms for assessing and rehabilitating elderly patients with functional and/or organic psychiatric illnesses. Data collected on service availability and training have provided guidelines for determining the range of community services needed, the number of hospital and long-term care beds required, and the personnel needed to be trained in psychogeriatrics (Royal College of Physicians and Royal College of Psychiatrists 1989; Wattis et al. 1981). Interpersonal collaboration between geriatricians and geriatric psychiatrists and between hospital-based and community-based staff servicing mentally ill elderly people provides a substantial opportunity to ensure continuity of care. Although, in theory, such collaboration is considered most desirable, it is not carried out routinely in practice.

The Netherlands

In a small country with a population of only 14.5 million people, of which 1.8 million (12.3%) are age 65 and over and 0.4 million (2.5%) are over age 80, psychogeriatrics itself has become a model of health care delivery. Psychiatric treatment and long-term clinical care, including nursing home care, are available to all who need it. Nursing homes recently have been placed under regional government control and, in the wake of long waiting periods for admission (6 months), services have been extended to support elderly people in their own homes. Recognizing the growing need for high-quality nursing home care in the country, the Royal Dutch Medical Association has approved a 2-year curriculum designed for physicians working in nursing homes. All 650 physicians now employed in nursing homes must be registered and certified. When additional facilities are constructed, high-quality, specially trained staff will be available immediately.

Psychosocial problems and dementia have been given priority for funding of research. A research budget of $13.5 million (U.S.) was allotted to a new 5-year national program to stimulate research on old age. Through this research, the Dutch hope to resolve another universal health care problem: the underdiagnosis of mental disorders in the elderly by primary care physicians. One major project at the Free University at Amsterdam is evaluating all older patients in 15 family practices, using screening instruments and diagnostic procedures for early diagnosis of dementia and differential diagnosis of dementia over the course of 4 years. The hoped-for product will be a diagnostic package through which primary care physicians can evaluate their older patients on a routine basis (Bleeker and Jonker 1990).

Though as yet underdeveloped in geriatric psychiatry, in the Netherlands, the integration of research and training with clinical practice has the potential to resolve two of the major problems currently prevalent in the practice of geriatric psychiatry.

Sweden

In Sweden, 17.4% of the total population are 65 years and over. Geriatric medicine has been rapidly expanding in primary care medicine as well as in specialties such as psychiatry (Bucht and Steen 1990). Other mental health professionals—nurses, psychologists, and social workers—and researchers in basic, clinical, epidemiological, and health services research have been drawn to the field as well.

In Sweden, apparently more so than in other countries, special programs have been established to enable small groups of patients with dementia to live in a milieu that is as homelike as possible (G. Bucht, P. O. Sandman, unpublished data, September 1990). Sixty such small group living arrangements were established in Sweden in 1987 alone. This type of living arrangement generally creates considerably less anxiety for the patient with dementia, provides better opportunities for social activities, and keeps the patient better oriented to reality. The desirability of private rooms is recognized as another means of maintaining patient autonomy for as long as possible. Trained personnel and continuous staff education and guidance can enhance the utility of these sheltered living group homes. Maintaining patients with dementia in the community in such a setting also reduces family caregiver burden and places less moral pressure on their relatives to visit the patient. Of a number of models ongoing in Sweden, this particular program was perhaps the most highly acclaimed. However, the inordinate cost of these services and high price paid by taxes as well as the difficulties encountered in maintaining staff education need to be taken into account.

An interesting study, underwritten and undertaken by a private foundation in collaboration with the medical faculty of the University of Göteborg, sought to determine whether older mentally ill patients function more appropriately in community-based home care or in long-term care facilities. Cognitive, functional, and needs assessments were carried out on a group of mentally ill elderly patients residing in nursing homes and a group cared for at home. Drug consumption and quality of life were also assessed and compared. When results were analyzed, the study found that the elderly patients who were able to affirm a choice of setting, whether home care or nursing home care, fared better than did patients who were unable to exercise the right to choose their care setting. The conclusions of this study are a major contribution toward the design of models of practice in both of these settings (Andersson 1989).

The high income tax paid in Sweden enables the development of unique health care services that cannot necessarily be duplicated elsewhere.

Switzerland

The organization of health care in Switzerland is not centralized. Switzerland does not have a centralized health and welfare ministry; rather, health care is decentralized among the country's 23 cantons. Each canton identifies and resolves the health care problems facing the indigenous elderly. The Task Force received a number of papers in English, German, French, and Italian describing a variety of psychogeriatric services.

As a whole, the needs of the elderly, whether residing in the home, nursing home, or hospitals, are being addressed at different levels of attention and intervention. For example, the emphasis in and near Lausanne, the Canton of Vaud, the urban hospital of Prilly, and the rural hospital of Gimel is on collaboration between geriatricians and geriatric psychiatrists (Wertheimer 1988). Generally, hospitalized patients receive specific rehabilitative services designed to arouse and support autonomy (Wertheimer 1985b, 1987). Other cantons emphasize other aspects of care, provide differing interventions, and utilize different combinations of professionals in care delivery.

Training in geriatric psychiatry is as varied as service delivery. No specific training program or duration of training is required for psychogeriatrics; few guidelines or mandates govern geriatric practice. Indeed, psychiatrists-in-training and other adult psychiatrists with a specialty interest in geriatric psychiatry may find themselves taken away from their elderly patients and urged to treat other age groups in the overall population. An assessment of the effectiveness of the current organization of psychogeriatric practice throughout Switzerland can be found in a publication by Wertheimer (1985a).

Israel

Israel is the only country in the world in which 90% of the elderly population were born elsewhere. The demographic changes that have taken place in Israel are also unique. The total population has increased from 600,000 in 1948 to over 3.6 million, excluding the most recent wave of immigrants from Russia and Ethiopia. The elderly population in other developed countries has doubled over four or five decades, whereas the elderly population of Israel has doubled in just two decades (Tropper 1990).

With the radical increase in the elderly population, a number of public and private organizations have become instrumental in assessing needs of the elderly and developing services and institutions to meet the growing need. The Ministry of Health has undertaken a study of needs of the elderly population and has recommended that a minimum of 2–5 beds per 1,000 persons age 65 and over be set in place. The Joint Distribution Committee, which originally established social shelters for the elderly, more recently has developed old age homes, special wards in general hospitals, and programs in community mental health centers and outpatient clinics targeted for the elderly. In 1974, the Joint Distribution Committee founded the Brookdale Institution of Gerontology and Adult Human Development in Jerusalem to engage in research planning and needs identification for the aged in Israel. This Center also addresses education and other relevant social issues in the field of aging. The results of the Center's applied research frequently lead to high-level policy-making decisions regarding the care and treatment of the elderly.

The Association for the Planning and Developing of Services for the Aged in Israel (ESHEL), working with the Joint Distribution Commission and the Ministries of Finance, Health and Labor and Social Affairs, supports a variety of community services and "progressive care models." Such models include acute inpatient and outpatient care, day care, long-term skilled nursing care, and community outreach programs. The Kupat-Holim, the health insurance institute of the general federation of labor to which the majority of medical institutions in the country belong, has demonstrated increased interest in enhancing existing geriatric and psychogeriatric services in the country. Based on an article by Tropper (1987), it appears that interest in psychogeriatrics, in particular, is advancing rapidly.

Japan

In Japan, as in other countries, there is a shortage of long-term care facilities. Care for elderly patients with dementia most often takes place in the home and is most often provided by relatives. Respite care and homemaker/chore services are difficult to arrange. In 1980, these problems led a group to organize an association of families caring for their elderly relatives with dementia. Its goal was to identify and resolve problems related to caregiving. In reality, self-support and advocacy appear to be the association's functions at the local level.

The Task Force's request for information bearing on specific models of care in Japan yielded only a paper describing recent developments in geriatric psychiatric research, focusing on epidemiology and clinical issues of age-associated dementia, especially that of caregiving (Hasegawa 1985; Homma and Hasegawa 1989). These authors are prolific writers, and many of their articles can be found in the Japanese and English literature.

In Summary

As we learn more about psychiatric services for the elderly in the United States and abroad, our ability to design model programs will advance. However, today's

Table 7. Population in millions, 1980–2000

	Total Pop.		Incr. %	Pop. 70+		Incr. %	Pop. 80+		Incr. %
(Total, aged 70+, 80+)	1980	2000		1980	2000		1980	2000	
Australia	14.5	17.8	23	0.8	1.3	58.7	0.2	0.3	61.4
Brazil	122.2	187.5	53	3.0	6.0	100	0.7	1.6	117.1
Egypt	42	64.4	53	0.8	1.7	112.5	0.1	0.3	146.9
France	53.5	56.3	5	5.1	5.6	10.4	1.4	1.5	4.9
Sweden	8.3	8.1	−2	0.9	1.0	11.1	0.2	0.3	36.9
Great Britain	55.9	55.2	−1	5.4	6.0	11.1	1.4	1.8	28.6
Japan	116.6	129.3	11	6.4	11.6	85.9	1.5	3.0	102.5
United States	223.2	236.8	18	15.6	20.6	32.1	4.4	5.8	31.8
Kenya	16.5	30.4	84	0.3	0.5	66.7	0.04	0.1	150.0
India	684.5	960.6	40	11.1	22.4	101.8	2.0	3.6	80.0

Source: Provisional projections of the United Population Division, New York, 1980; adapted from Andersson 1989 with permission.

capacity to meet the mental health needs of our global aging population cannot match that population's growth (Table 7).

Although the proportion of older persons varies from nation to nation, it is clear that the greatest increase in the population over 70 years of age is yet to come for many countries. As less developed nations gray, new innovations in care delivery must surely be designed. Much can be learned from our work to date; much remains to be learned in the future.

Chapter 8

Problems and Recommendations

Although access to and availability of community-based mental health services for the elderly are largely Medicare driven, care opportunities in long-term nursing homes are Medicaid driven. Dependence on these two insurance mechanisms poses considerable difficulties for the psychiatric care of patients with dementia, or otherwise mentally impaired or emotionally disturbed elderly. While a variety of psychogeriatric models of care have established both their usefulness and effectiveness, the mental health problems of the elderly and their families require considerably more resources than have been made available to date. As our aging population increases, the magnitude of the problem will only increase.

Problem 1

Treatment models in geriatric psychiatry, albeit limited in number, are innovative and solve unique problems confronting elderly mentally ill people. Yet, despite their effectiveness, these models do not tend to be replicated in many other sites. Some needs of mentally ill elderly people are geographically determined, differing in rural, suburban, and urban settings. Thus, exemplary programs often are not accessible, available, or affordable to many of our nation's elderly.

Recommendations

✦ The American Psychiatric Association's Board of Trustees should give consideration to the establishment of a *Committee on the Practice of Geriatric Psychiatry under the Council on Aging.* A formal charge has been developed. Such a committee should function in close collaboration with APA components on education, ethnic minorities, the public and private sectors, long-term care, public affairs, professional activities, and biographical surveys. The Agency for

Health Care Policy and Research (AHCPR), the National Center for Health Statistics (NCHS), and other organizations and agencies could become a resource to such a committee.

✦ Federal funding agencies, including the recently created AHCPR, should give high priority to well-designed short- and long-term outcome studies of specialty assessment and treatment programs for mentally ill elderly people. Such studies would facilitate greater collaboration among clinicians, researchers, and data analysts in this important area.

✦ The NCHS should begin to specify in its health surveys and reports of findings whether mental health services received by the elderly were provided by specialty service programs with specialty staff. Moreover, the NCHS should maintain a data base on the availability and growth of these specialty services.

✦ The APA's Office of Public Affairs, working with the Council on Aging, should initiate a special program for both consumers and providers to help destigmatize mental health care for the elderly and their families.

Problem 2

Primary care physicians and other physicians utilized by the community-based elderly for physical health care problems frequently overlook, trivialize, or ignore the need for mental health intervention for the elderly and their families. Primary care physicians rarely implement timely or appropriate assessment or referral of their older patients and families for mental health intervention.

Recommendations

✦ Outreach efforts should be undertaken by the APA to work with the American Academy of Family Practitioners and the American College of Physicians to improve primary care physician evaluation and referral of the elderly and families with mental health problems.

✦ Continuing medical education for primary care physicians should place emphasis on the recognition, treatment, and referral of psychopathology of late life. The current primary care geriatric education research study underway in the Netherlands may provide insight into an alternative mechanism through which education for those in primary care practice may be provided.

✦ Ongoing development and expansion of divisions of geriatric psychiatry within departments of psychiatry will broaden the base of clinicians able to provide state-of-the-art clinical care to older patients and their families, able to serve as models and consultants to other physicians, and able to train medical students, residents, and fellows.

✦ The APA and other organizations should advocate the resumption of federally supported fellowships in geriatric psychiatry to increase the number of clinicians, teachers, and researchers in geriatric psychiatry.

✦ To foster greater knowledge of the special physical and mental health care needs of the elderly, residents in psychiatry, internal medicine, and family practice should be required to take rotations in geriatric psychiatry programs. Psychiatry residency training and psychiatrists' continuing medical education should include greater emphasis on issues of prevention, assessment, and treatment of elder abuse, neglect, and exploitation.

Problem 3

Medicare reimbursement has provided economic disincentives to the mental health treatment of the elderly for both the patient and the psychiatrist. As structured, until January 1992, the treatment of the elderly and their families in outpatient and community outreach settings and in nursing homes has been discouraged. Outpatient and nursing home psychiatric treatment has been restricted by the imposition of a unique 50% patient-borne copayment; inpatient psychiatric care has been subject to a 1-day deductible for each care episode, and a 190-day lifetime limit. Regional variances prevailed; coinsurance payments were unpredictable.

Recommendations

✦ The Health Care Financing Administration needs to mandate nationally uniform interpretation of Evaluation/Management (E/M) Current Procedural Terminology (CPT) codes for all medical specialists with penalties to regional carriers for noncompliance.

✦ Reimbursement with 20% copayment need to be established regardless of location of service.

✦ The Medigap issue needs to be resolved in favor of older persons who have private health insurance that supplements Medicare. The elderly need assurance that secondary insurers pay Medicare deductibles and copayments.

✦ Medical reimbursement policies are too restrictive and create a severe financial disincentive for psychiatrists to have an appropriate proportion of their practice in geriatric psychiatry when there are not enough psychiatrists to begin with and practices could well be filled with younger patients for whom reimbursement is relatively less restrictive and who do have the option to pay private fees at rates agreed upon between doctor and patient.

Problem 4

The universal bottleneck confronting those seeking access to nursing home care has led to overburdened family caregivers who lack for community health and service support when a patient is discharged from an acute care facility to the home to await nursing home placement. For other patients and families, the same bottleneck also has resulted in the inappropriate retention of chronically mentally and physically ill elderly patients in acute care hospitals while awaiting nursing home beds.

Recommendations

✦ The availability of affordable and accessible community-based respite resources should be improved. Such facilities both "normalize" the lives of caregivers and enhance the quality of life for dementia patients or elderly people who are otherwise mentally impaired.

✦ Home health care should be expanded to include well-trained home mental health care personnel who are brought together with the patient and family caregivers prior to the patient's discharge from the hospital. Ongoing training and incentives should be set in place to encourage personnel retention in these important jobs.

✦ Adequate federal support should be provided to states to support the capacity of adult protective services to intervene on behalf of older individuals with dementia and their caregivers when necessary.

✦ APA could ensure attention to mental health issues by working with the Administration on Aging in the development of its Elder Care Institutes, whose charge is to help identify the needs of elderly people in the community and develop in-home and community-based elder care.

✦ Federally funded needs assessment for institutional beds with appropriate staffing patterns is in order. A projection of bed needs over the next several decades and establishment of humane institutional settings that provide a high quality of life for residents are both overdue.

Problem 5

Although models of geriatric psychiatry programs have been developed within the Veterans Administration (VA) system, they remain the exception rather than the rule.

Recommendation

✦ Just as Congress mandated special service programs within the VA for posttraumatic stress disorder and substance abuse, so too Congress should mandate that psychogeriatric programs be made a specific priority within the VA system to meet the needs of the aging veteran and his or her family.

Problem 6

The APA Professional Activities and Biographical Directory Survey requests psychiatrists to specify the percentage of patients age 65 and over carried in their practice and the settings in which they see them. No data are collected on the time spent with older patients and their families as a proportion of total work time. The level of specialty training is not solicited; no information about relative reimbursement received is collected.

Recommendations

✦ In the next APA Professional Activities Survey, this Task Force recommends that data be collected on time spent with elderly patients, their families, and other informal or formal care providers. Actual reimbursement received per unit of time should be collected and analyzed. Time spent needs to be divided by tasks performed. Instead of defining "specialists" by the numbers of elderly patients served, "specialists" should be identified by the nature of training, specialty qualifications, or their equivalent. This is vital information for effective enlightenment of policymakers and changes in reimbursement patterns.

✦ Research questions for the survey should be submitted by members of the Council on Aging.

References

American Psychiatric Association, Office of Economic Affairs: A Review of the Extent and Trends in Insurance Coverage for Psychiatric Illness in the Private Sector, Based on the Annual Bureau of Labor Statistics Level of Benefit Studies. Washington DC, American Psychiatric Association, 1985

American Psychiatric Association: Diagnostic and Statistical Manual of Mental Disorders. Washington, DC, American Psychiatric Association, 1987

Andersson M: Elderly Patients in Nursing Homes and in Homecare: Scope of Institutional Care, Characteristics, Motor and Intellectual Functions, Drug Consumption and Quality of Life. Göteborg, Sweden, Vasastadens Bokbinderi AB, 1989

Arie T: Some current issues in old age psychiatry, in The Provision of Mental Health Services in Britain. Edited by Wilkinson G, Freeman H. London, England, Royal College of Psychiatrists, 1986, pp 79–89

Arie T, Jolley D: Making services work: organization and style of psychiatric services, in The Psychiatry of Late Life. Edited by Levy R, Post F. Boston, MA, Blackwell Scientific Publications, 1982, pp 222–251

Barsa JJ, Kass F, Beels CC, et al: Development of a cost-efficient psychogeriatric services. Am J Psychiatry 142:238–241, 1985

Berger S, King E: Designing services for the elderly. AORN Journal 51:2, 1990

Bienenfeld D, Wheeler BG: Psychiatric services to nursing home: a liaison model. Hosp Community Psychiatry 40:793–794, 1989

Billig N, Leibenluft E: Special considerations in integrating elderly patients into a general hospital psychiatry unit. Hosp Community Psychiatry 38:3, 1987

Blalock R, Dial TH: Psychiatry and the Elderly: A Preliminary Analysis of Differences in Practitioner Characteristics (NIMH Report 8 5-M043907301D). Rockville, MD, National Institute of Mental Health, 1982

Bleeker JAC, Jonker C: Status of psychogeriatrics in the Netherlands. International Psychogeriatrics 2:169–173, 1990

Borson S, Liptzin B, Nininger J, et al: Psychiatry and the nursing home. Am J Psychiatry 144(11):1412–1418, 1987

Borson S, Liptzin B, Nininger J, et al: Nursing Homes and the Mentally Ill Elderly: A Report of the Task Force on Nursing Homes and the Mentally Ill Elderly. Washington, DC, American Psychiatric Association, 1989

Bucht G, Steen B: Development of psychogeriatric medicine in Sweden. International Psychogeriatrics 2:73–80, 1990

Burns BJ, Taube CA: Mental health services in general medical care and in nursing homes, in Mental Health Policy for Older Americans: Protecting Minds at Risk. Edited by Fogel BS, Furino A, Gottlieb G. Washington DC, American Psychiatric Press, 1990, pp 63–84

Bush CT, Langford MW, Rosen P, et al: Operation outreach: intensive case management for severely psychiatrically disabled adults. Hosp Community Psychiatry 41:647–649, 1990

Butler RN: Why Survive? Growing Old in America. New York, Harper & Row, 1975

Cohen C: Integrated community services, in Comprehensive Review of Geriatric Psychiatry. Edited by Sadavoy J, Lazarus LW, Jarvik LF. Washington DC, American Psychiatric Press, 1991, pp 613–634

Cohen GD: The interface of mental and physical health phenomena in later life: new directions in geriatric psychiatry. Gerontology and Geriatrics Education 9:3, 1989

Conwell Y, Nelson JC, Kim K, et al: Elderly patients admitted to the psychiatric unit of a general hospital. J Am Geriatr Soc 37:35–41, 1989

Copeland JRM: Organization of services for the elderly mentally, in Handbook of Studies of Psychiatry and Old Age. Edited by Kay DW, Burrows GD. Amsterdam, Netherlands, Elsevier, 1984, pp 485–506

Copeland JRM, Gurland BJ: International comparative studies, in Recent Advances in Psychogeriatrics. Edited by Arie T. New York, Churchill, Livingstone, 1985, pp 175–195

Department of Veterans Affairs: Report on Treatment of the Geriatric Psychiatric Patient. Washington, DC, Mental Health and Behavioral Sciences Service, Department of Veterans Affairs, 1982

Department of Veterans Affairs: Summary of Medical Programs. Washington, DC, Office of Information and Analysis (742), Department of Veterans Affairs, 1990

Department of Veterans Affairs: Integrated Psychiatric Care: Guidelines, Criteria and Standards (Circular 10-91-32). Washington, DC, Department of Veterans Affairs, Veterans Health Care and Research Administration, 1991

Fogel BS, Colenda C, deFigueiredo JM, et al: State Mental Hospitals and the Elderly: A Task Force Report of the American Psychiatric Association. Washington, DC, American Psychiatric Association (in press)

Folstein MF, Folstein SE, McHugh PR: Mini-Mental State: a practical method for grading the cognitive state of patients for the clinician. J Psychiatr Res 12:189–198, 1975

Ford C, Sbordane R: Attitudes of psychiatrists towards elderly patients. Am J Psychiatry 137:571–575, 1980

Ford CV, Spar JE, Davis B, et al: Hospital treatment of elderly neuropsychiatric patients, I: initial clinical and administrative experience with a new teaching ward. J Am Geriatr Soc 28:446–450, 1980

Franklin JL, Solovitz B, Mason M: An evaluation of case management. Am J Public Health 77:674–678, 1987

Gallagher RM, McCann WJ, Jerman A, et al: The behavioral medicine service; an administrative model for biopsychosocial medical care, teaching and research. Gen Hosp Psychiatry 12:283–295, 1990

German PS, Shapiro S, Skinner EA, et al: Detection and management of mental health problems of older patients by primary care providers. JAMA 257:489–493, 1987

Glasscote RM, Gudeman JE, Miles DG: Creative Mental Health Services for the Elderly. Washington DC, Joint Information Service of the American Psychiatric Association and the Mental Health Association, 1977

Goldberg RL: Geriatric consultation/liaison psychiatry (Issues in Geriatric Psychiatry). Adv Psychosom Med 19:138–150, 1989

Goldstein MZ: Evaluation of the elderly patient, in Verwoerdt's Clinical Geropsychiatry. Edited by Bienenfeld D. Baltimore, MD, Williams & Wilkins, 1990, pp 47–57

Gottlieb G: Financial issues affecting psychiatric care of the elderly. Paper presented at the first annual conference on Current Issues in Geriatric Psychiatry, SUNY Buffalo School of Medicine and Biomedical Sciences Department of Psychiatry and the Western New York Geriatric Education Center, Buffalo, NY, April 1988

Greene JA, Asp J: The geriatric patient: a creative practice approach. J Tenn Med Assoc 79:77–81, 1986

Greenhill MH, Kilgore SR: Principles of methodology in teaching the psychiatric approach to medical house officers. Psychosom Med 12:38–38, 1950

Greenhill MH: Models of liaison programs that address age and cultural differences in reaction to illness. Bibiotecha Psychiatrica 159:77–81, 1979

Hasegawa K: The epidemiological study on psychogeriatric disorders in Japan. Proceedings of the International Symposium on Psychiatric Epidemiology, 1985, pp 301–312

Heltman LR, Adler NE: The Aging Veteran Population: Implications for VA Health Care Services. Washington, DC, Management Sciences Service, Department of Veterans Affairs, 1990

Hemsi L: Psychogeriatric care in the community, in The Psychiatry of Late Life. Edited by Levy R, Post F. Boston, MA, Blackwell Scientific, 1982, 252–287

Homma A, Hasegawa, K: Recent developments in gerontopsychiatric research on age associated dementia in Japan. International Psychogeriatrics 1:31–49, 1989

Intagliata J: Improving the quality of community care for the chronically mentally disabled: the role of case management. Schizophr Bull 8:655–674, 1982

Jencks SF: Recognition of mental distress and diagnosis of mental disorders in primary care. JAMA 253:1903–1097, 1985

Kantor J: Clinical case management: definition, principles and components. Hosp Community Psychiatry 40:361–368, 1989

Kay DWK, Roth M, Hall MRP: Special problems of the aged and the organization of hospital services. BMJ 2:967–972, 1966

Kiloh LG: Pseudo-dementia. Acta Psychiatr Scand 37:336–351, 1961

Klein JI, Macbeth JE, Noek J: Legal Issues in the Private Practice of Psychiatry. Washington, DC, American Psychiatric Press, 1984

Koran LM: Medical-psychiatric units and the future of psychiatric practice. Psychosomatics 26:171–175, 1985

Koran LM: The Nation's Psychiatrists. Washington, DC, American Psychiatric Association, 1987

Lebowitz BD, Light E, Bailey F: Mental health center services for the elderly: the impact of coordination with area agencies on aging. Gerontologist 27:699–702, 1987

Light E, Lebowitz BD, Bailey F: CMHCs and elderly services: an analysis of direct and indirect services and service delivery sites. Community Ment Health J 22:294–302, 1986

Lippert GP, Conn D, Schogt B, et al: Psychogeriatric consultation: general hospital versus home for the aged. Gen Hosp Psychiatry 12:313–318, 1990

Lipowski Z: The need to integrate liaison psychiatry and geropsychiatry. Am J Psychiatry 140:1003–1005, 1983

McKegney FP, Schwartz CE: Behavioral medicine: treatment and organizational issues. Gen Hosp Psychiatry 8:330–339, 1986

Milazzo-Sayre LJ, Benson PR, Rosenstein MJ, et al: Use of Inpatient Psychiatric Services by the Elderly Age 65 and Over, U.S. 1980 (Mental Health Statistical Note No 181). Rockville, MD, U.S. Department of Health and Human Services—ADAMHA-NIMH, Division of Biometry and Applied Sciences Survey and Reports Branch, April 1987

Mohl PC: The liaison psychiatrist: social role and status. Pychosomatics 20:19–23, 1979

National Center for Health Statistics: Utilizing short-stay hospitals (Annual Survey for the United States, 1980: Ser B, No 64). Washington, DC, U.S. Department of Health and Human Service, 1982

Norman A: Mental illness in old age: meeting the challenge, in Policy Studies in Aging No 1, Centre for Policy on Aging. Dorset, England, Dorset Press, 1980

Parish BV, Landsberg G: Developing a geriatric mental health outreach unit in a rural community. Journal of Geriatric Social Work 7:75–82, 1984

Perez E, Silverman M, Blouin B: Psychiatric consultation to elderly medical and surgical inpatients in a general hospital. Psychiatr Q 57:18–22, 1985

Pfeiffer E: A Short Portable Mental Status Questionnaire for the Assessment of Organic Brain Deficit in Elderly Patients. J Am Geriatr Soc 23:433–441, 1975

Pfeiffer E, Johnson TM, Chiofolo RC: Functional assessment of elderly subjects in four service settings. Paper presented at the Annual Scientific meeting, Gerontological Society of America, San Diego, CA, November 21–25, 1980

Popkin M, Mackensie T, Callies A: Psychiatric consultation to geriatric medically ill inpatients in a university hospital. Arch Gen Psychiatry 41:703–707, 1984

Rapp SR, Paris S, Wallace CE: Comorbid psychiatric disorders in elderly medical patients: a 1 year prospective study. J Am Geriatr Soc 39:124–141, 1991

Raschko R: Program Report: Elderly Services—A Multidisciplinary In-home Evaluation, Treatment and Case Management Program. Spokane, WA, Spokane Community Mental Health Center, 1987

Reifler, BV, Kathely A, O'Neill P, et. al: Five-year experience of a community outreach program for the elderly. Am J Psychiatry 139:220–223, 1982

Rosse R, Ciolino C, Gurel L: Utilization of psychiatric consultation with an elderly medically ill inpatient population in a VA hospital. Milit Med 151:583–586, 1986

Royal College of Physicians and the Royal College of Psychiatrists: Care of Elderly People with Mental Illness: Specialist Services and Medical Training. London, England, The Royal College of Physicians of London and The Royal College of Psychiatrists, 1989

Royal College of Psychiatrists/British Geriatric Society: Guidelines for collaboration between geriatric physicians and psychiatrists in the care of the elderly. Bulletin of the Royal College of Psychiatrists, November 1979, pp 168–169

Rubenstein, LZ, Abrass IB, Kane RL: The role of geriatric assessment units in caring for the elderly: an analytic review. J Am Geriatr Soc 28:539–543, 1980

Rubenstein LZ, Abrass IB, Kane RL: Improved care for patients on a new geriatric evaluation unit. J Am Geriatr Soc 29:531–536, 1982a

Rubenstein LZ, Rhee L, Kane RL: The role of geriatric assessment units in caring for the elderly: An analytic review. J Gerontology 37:513–521, 1982b

Ruskin P: Geropsychiatric consultation in a university hospital: a report on 67 referrals. Am J Psychiatry 142:333–336, 1985

Sakauye KM, Baker FM, Jimenez R, et al: Report of the Task Force on Ethnic Minority Elderly: A Task Force Report of the American Psychiatric Association. Washington, DC, American Psychiatric Association (in press)

Schurman RA, Kramer PD, Mitchell JB: The hidden mental health network. Arch Gen Psychiatry 42:89–94, 1985

Schwartz C, Stove T, Bennet M: Treatment of the elderly on a general hospital psychiatric short-stay unit. Can J Psychiatry 25:633–637, 1980

Shapiro S, Kinner EA, Kramer M, et al: Measuring need for mental health services in a general population. Med Care 23:1033–1043, 1985

Small G, Fawzy F: Psychiatric consultation for the medically ill elderly in the general hospital: need for a collaborative model of care. Psychosomatics 29:94–103, 1988

Stein L: Comments by Leonard Stein. Hosp Community Psychiatry 41:649–651, 1990

Stein EM: Community-based psychiatric ambulatory care: the private practice model, in Psychiatry and Old Age: An International Text. Edited by Copeland J, Blazer D, Abou-Saleh M. Sussex, England, Wiley (in press)

Stein SR, Linn MW, Edelstein J, et al: Elderly patients satisfaction with care under HMO versus private systems. South Med J 82:3–8, 1989

Strain JJ, Pincus HA, Houpt JL, et al: Models of mental health training for primary care physicians. Psychosom Med 47:95–110, 1985

Strain JJ, Lyons JS, Hammer JS, et al: Cost offset from a psychiatric consultation-liaison intervention with elderly hip fracture patients. Am J Psychiatry 148:1044–1049, 1991

Thompson KS, Griffith EEH, Leaf PJ: A historical review of the Madison model of community care. Hosp Community Psychiatry 41:625–634, 1990

Tropper MS: Psychogeriatric medicine in Israel. The International Psychogeriatric Association Newsletter 4:7–11, 1987

Tropper MS: Psychogeriatrics in Israel: present and future. International Psychogeriatrics 2:175–177, 1990

Wattis J, Wattis L, Arie T: Psychogeriatrics: a national survey of a new branch of psychiatry. BMJ 282:1959–1633, 1981

Wertheimer J: Evaluation of effectiveness of a psycho-geriatric sector organization, in Psychiatry, Vol 5. Edited by Pichot P, Berner P, Wolf R, et al. New York, Plenum, 1985a, pp 437–441

Wertheimer J: Animation dans les services de psychogeriatrie. La Revue de Geriatrie 10:315–318, 1985b

Wertheimer J: Rehabilitation and long-term care in the elderly, in Psychogeriatrics: An International Handbook. Edited by Bergener M. New York, Springer, 1987, pp 407–431

Wertheimer J: Organisation des soins psychogeriatriques: principes et applications. Moderne Geriatrie 10:41–50, 1988

Yesavage J, Brink J, Rose T, et al: Development and validation of a geriatric screening scale: a preliminary report. J Psychiatr Res 17:37–49, 1983

Young LD, Harsch H: Inpatient unit for combined physical and psychiatric disorders. Psychosomatics 27:53–60, 1980

Index

Page numbers printed in **boldface** *type refer to tables or figures.*

Activities of daily living, assistance with, 16, 19, **19**, 47
Adapted Work Program (AWP), of Geriatric Research, Education, and Clinical Center, 33
Administration on Aging, Elder Care Institutes of, 64
Adult day program, 16
  of Baycrest Center comprehensive geriatric psychiatry care program, 49–50
  of Geriatric Psychiatry Program (West Los Angeles, CA), 34
Adult protective services, need for, 64
Age, of psychiatrists working with geriatric population, 40
Alcohol, Drug Abuse and Mental Health Administration (ADAMHA), 54
American Academy of Family Practitioners, need for APA outreach to, 62
American College of Physicians, need for APA outreach to, 62
American Psychiatric Association (APA)
  need for advocacy of funding for training by, 63

need for establishment of committee on geriatric psychiatry by, 61–62
need for outreach to primary care physicians by, 62
professional activities and biographical directory survey conducted by, 39–44
Apartment program, of Baycrest Center comprehensive geriatric psychiatry care program, 47
Area Agencies on Aging (AAAs)
  CMHC relationships with, 10–11
  funding provided by, 17
Assertive Continuous Care Teams (ACCT), 11
Assessment, in inpatient psychogeriatric unit, 24
Association for the Planning and Developing of Services for the Aged in Israel (ESHEL), 58

Baycrest Center, 45–51
  Department of Psychiatry at, 48–50
  philosophy and services of, 46–48
Baycrest Center comprehensive geriatric psychiatry care model, 45–51